SOUL SOARING

NEW TECHNIQUES FOR DIAGNOSING AND OVERCOMING
WHAT SEPARATES YOU FROM HARMONY WITHIN

About the Author

Mary Clement completed a dual degree in law and social work (JD/MSW), and earned her Ph.D. in sociology, at Washington State University in Pullman. She is a practicing counselor, and also currently is an associate professor in the Department of Criminal Justice at Virginia Commonwealth University in Richmond. There, she coordinates a dual degree program between VCU and the School of Theology of Virginia Union University, or Union Theological Seminary in Virginia, that offers a Master of Divinity and a Master of Science in Criminal Justice. Her published body of work includes textbooks and articles that deal with law enforcement and corrections, women in prisons, and troubled and abused youth in the juvenile justice system.

SOUL SOARING

NEW TECHNIQUES FOR DIAGNOSING AND OVERCOMING
WHAT SEPARATES YOU FROM HARMONY WITHIN

BY

MARY CLEMENT, PH.D.

THE OAKLEA PRESS
RICHMOND, VIRGINIA

FIRST EDITION
First Printing, August, 1998

SOUL SOARING, New Techniques for Diagnosing and Overcoming What Separates You from Harmony Within, Printed in the United States of America. For information write The Oaklea Press, P. O. Box 29334, Richmond, Virginia 23242-0334.

ISBN 1-892538-17-2

PREFACE

During the twenty-five years that I have spent teaching in various universities, I've awaken to my spiritual nature. But this awakening did not come without difficulty. You see, I was trained as a research scientist with a Ph.D. in sociology. Because of my training, I viewed the possibility of an unseen reality with skepticism. As a result, my spiritual unfolding came slowly, and in stages.

It first began when I decided to explore my Native American heritage, and to participate in the practice of some of the traditions of my father's fathers. This began two decades ago when I was living in Wichita, Kansas, and teaching at the state university. A woman who operated a health food store had a private practice of massage and body reflexology, and I became her patient. She was working on the tightness in my neck. I was lying on the table, and noticed a flash of light so bright it was as though lightning had struck the building.

"Is there a storm outside?" I asked.

"No," she replied.

"But I saw a flash of light."

She explained that when she was working on a patient and needed guidance from another realm, she would put up a silent prayer. In answer to it, she would see a flash of light or would hear a ringing sound. This confirmed the location that most needed her attention. She'd been expecting the light, but was surprised I'd seen it.

I visited this woman several times. One day she said that my high cheekbones and wide pelvis indicated I must be a Cherokee (a member of an Iroquois-speaking tribe of North America), like herself. She wondered if I would like to go to a local Indian powwow, an event, she explained, that might be compared to a dance.

My curiosity had been aroused, and I agreed. Off we went on a warm summer evening in her car to a rural area comprised mostly of wheat fields. She turned off the highway onto a dirt road and, finally, into a cow pasture. A small grove of trees protected people from the hot Kansas sun. There I saw men dressed in blue jeans, cotton short-sleeved shirts, cowboy hats and boots. They stood around talking to one other, some leaning against their late model cars and pickup trucks. The women were dressed just as simply, for the most part in laborers' clothes. Their long, straight hair and dark features indicated to me that these were the real people of the plains. Strangely, I felt at home.

I don't remember everything about that night, but I do recall the friend who brought me greeting the others and introducing me around. They seemed to approve of my being there. In a short time some men began beating on a large drum. Their voices created a kind of singing chant, unlike anything I'd ever heard. The atmosphere was transformed as if by magic. Men and women danced together in a single circle, everyone moving in one direction.

Next, the women danced alone. They formed a circle, each moving her feet in a slow, two-step motion. Then my friend did something that changed my life. She put her shawl over my arm and gently pushed me into the middle, where I danced, the other women encircling me. It was, I realized, an initiation. When an Indian maiden first dances with a shawl, the rite of passage from childhood into the society of women is recognized. Later, I learned that for a shawl to be given to a woman for this first dance is a special honor.

For me it was more than a rite of passage, it was an opening of my heart and of buried memories. It is not too much to say that I experienced a shift in my consciousness. Suddenly, I became aware of and sensitive to the spirits of Native Americans, present and past. This new sensitivity improved the quality of my life, my inner harmony and the effectiveness of my teaching. My sensitivity grew further after I moved to Virginia. I had strange and wonderful experiences when I came upon sacred Indian lands and graves, and was able to help trapped Indian spirits walk into the light.

Another period of accelerated growth came while I was studying for a dual degree in social work and law. In the social work program students were encouraged to go through therapy themselves in order to better understand the different therapies. In doing so, I gained a better understanding of myself. My studies expanded into family therapy, and I became more enlightened about family systems. As my awareness grew, unusual experiences and coincidences seemed to take place more frequently, and the clarity of my consciousness became heightened. In one instance I went away on a two-week retreat to work intensely with a therapist, and found that the therapist and clients had created their own dysfunctional family. The women worked hard to cover for the men. I began to see this as a "laboratory experiment" that enhanced what I'd been learning in books and the sessions with my family therapist.

At this retreat I met two English women who could heal with their hands. I was amazed to find that their hands became hot with energy. They taught me how to meditate and how to connect in a way that allowed me, too, to send energy of light with hands that became hot. This retreat was a first episode of what I have come to call "cover." Cover is when I go somewhere or do something thinking that it is for one purpose, but in reality, God has another purpose, and a far more important lesson to teach.

My growth was having a profound and positive impact on my practice. Then one day, a friend came to me who was struggling to decide whether or not to leave her abusive husband. Rather than work with her in my office, I led her to a quiet spot that had meaning for me. Perhaps here, I thought, she would be able to get in touch with her inner needs and true desires. Instead, she taught me a profound lesson.

Before that day I'd never seriously entertained the possibility of past lives. I'd had doubts, of course — moments when past lives seemed possible — but I'd always dismissed those feelings out of hand. For me, this life was the only one.

The place I'd taken her was sacred Indian land. There, to my astonishment, my friend experienced flashes of memories of a life spent as an American Indian. These memories made her fearful and disturbed. She said that she recalled leaving her tribe and, as a result, facing death.

Aside from wondering about the validity of these memory flashes, I wondered why a fear of death would be associated with the act of leaving today. Then it came to me. This belief would have been true for an Indian woman of long ago. An individual attempting to live alone in the wilderness without the help and support of others would have faced great difficulty, and probably would not have survived very long. If these past lives indeed had existed, it seemed logical that the fear of separation would continue to resonate in this life.

Her old beliefs about leaving and dying no longer were consistent with the reality of her situation. But nevertheless the belief was there, buried beneath the surface. It would have to be canceled out somehow, and replaced with a new belief in concert with the circumstances of today. This idea of buried memories, perhaps from the collective unconscious or from previous lives, was what I learned about that day, and I began to incorporate this into my counseling practice.

Let me make it clear that it is not the goal of this book, nor is it within the scope of what will be written here, to prove that reincarnation is a fact. It is true, of course, that a belief in reincarnation is held by a majority of the world's population, and that compelling evidence has surfaced in recent years that supports the possibility. But this does not make it so beyond the shadow of a doubt. Other plausible explanations can be promulgated for what my friend experienced. Many, both in and out of the scientific community, have hypothesized that only one Universal Mind exists, and that each of us is connected to this Universal Unconscious Mind through our own individual subconscious mind.

The psychiatrist Carl Jung, for example, upon observing the dreams of patients and studying the world's mythology and religious literature, concluded that there must exist universal psychic patterns called *archetypes.* He said these archetypes live within a Universal Mind, or a *Collective Unconscious,* as he called it. According to Jung, these archetype patterns govern both the forms of nature and the experiences and behaviors of human beings.

The biologist Rupert Sheldrake, in his books *New Science of Life* and *The Presence of the Past,* argues a similar theme. He presents extensive evidence to show how both the forms and laws of nature are the result of life energy being patterned by invisible force fields. Like ideas existing in another dimension, these *morphogenetic* force fields, as Sheldrake calls them, are the reason a particular plant or animal assumes its given shape and displays its particular characteristics or behavior.

What these influential theories, from a psychiatrist and a

biologist, have in common is that they both state that ideas are real in and of themselves. Ideas exist in another dimension. They're the underlying reality that become the original causes of what we experience in the visible, physical world. Ideas have their effect through their patterns. Ideas create physical reality. Ideas create our own individual and unique reality as well.

Perhaps my friend tapped into, or tuned into, the portion of the Collective Unconscious that houses memories of fear and death associated with abandonment. Perhaps her personal morphogenetic field is part of a larger morphogenetic field shared by Native Americans, and so the memories of that race are contained within it. Another, similar theory suggests that as a descendant of American Indians, her DNA contains the collective memory and conditioning of generations who have gone before. In either case her fear of separation might be viewed as a kind of instinct, which had been programmed in.

A more traditional view would hold that reading or learning that took place in this lifetime caused the beliefs to be lodged in her subconscious. But in my view, how they got there is not the most important issue, nor necessarily relevant to her liberation from their debilitating effect. What's important is that her fear was real. Our visit to the burial ground somehow triggered anxiety that came from beliefs that needed to be examined and modified in order to be consistent with today's reality.

For now, let us return to the review of what led to a period in my life of accelerated personal growth. Study in social work brought about part of it. Law school and the process leading there brought profound changes in me as well, and for strange reasons. To begin with, I had a hard time getting in because I had difficulty scoring above the thirtieth percentile on the entrance examination (LSAT). After performing poorly five times in a row, I underwent testing and was found to have a learning disability. As a result, I went to a therapist who had a practice which had been inspired by Paul Dennison's work with learning-disabled children.

First, we addressed the emotional aspects of the disability. Then I learned and practiced physical exercises such as the cross-crawl. In this exercise a person stands and touches her right hand to her left leg, then the left hand to the right leg, while simultaneously humming. At the same time the individual moves her eyes to the left, to the right, then up and down. The objective of all this motion is to open up the brain and have it working in its entirety. When a person's brain has been re-patterned to enable her to simultaneously access both right and left sides of the brain, the individual can more fully employ the power of the right brain, which is the storehouse of memory.

All sorts of connections became apparent between the psychotherapies I had been studying and this new approach, which also included a technique called kinesiology. That involves testing the strength or weakness of muscles in certain situations. Chiropractors already were using kinesiology to find out which parts of the body needed realignment. What I learned was that the technique could be used to provide clues to a person's subconscious beliefs. For example, if I had asked my friend before we visited the Indian burial ground whether she believed that leaving her husband could result in her death, her answer would have been a resounding "No." This is because her conscious beliefs were in line with today's reality.

Suppose, however, that she agreed to answer a series of "yes" or "no" questions, while holding the thumb and forefinger of her right hand together tightly. To perform this procedure, I would take her thumb in one of my hands and her forefinger in the other, and tell her to hold them tight. But her muscles would involuntarily relax — and I'd be able to pull them apart easily — if a subconscious belief existed in opposition to what she consciously held to be true.

Now suppose that I held her thumb and forefinger in this manner and asked a series of questions. If I asked about a fear of separation, her muscles would have relaxed no matter how adamantly she insisted that no such belief existed. I'd then have been able to track down the source of the problem by asking questions that eventually would have lead to the time the fear had been formed (in ancient American Indian times).

So what I learned because of my disability and my desire to enter law school was that kinesiology (muscle testing) could be used to identify specific problems that my clients needed to work on in therapy sessions. I was able to test the effectiveness of kinesiology/results therapy in my practice and later used it extensively with women in prison. In those sessions most of the therapy focused on childhood, because the inmates had experienced so much trauma.

In 1993 I began to work with a woman I'll call Pearl. (She and the other clients I discuss in these pages have been given pseudonyms to protect their privacy.) Though Pearl was my patient, she also became my teacher as we together explored dimensions not covered in my training as a social worker. Not only did my knowledge expand during that time, but many of my colleagues also experienced memories of past lives, or parts of past lives (or perhaps they tapped into the collective unconscious or the morphogenetic field of their family group, if you prefer one of those explanations) — using kinesiology/results therapy.

Traditionally, as you may know, regression therapy has been conducted by means of hypnosis, and a drawback is that patients don't always remember what they experience. By contrast kinesiology's self-regression therapy enables people to remember and to fully experience feelings brought to the surface by memories. The therapy parts the veil that covers them, thereby illuminating the causes of present-day stress. It provides a means to move quickly to a higher level of understanding. This often results in people making changes in their lives that rapidly result in tangible benefits. Those who have been stuck for years, for example, or who have been reluctant to change, often suddenly shed long-buried fears. Because they now understand the root of a problem or irrational belief, they often can more easily muster the courage to move forward and leave encumbering emotional baggage behind.

As my clients and I became exposed to a larger reality dwelling within us, we began to have experiences with higher beings. In my case I was aware at first of some greater force of energy, like an angel. This force would be present when someone was conducting kinesiology on me. Soon I realized that the angel could come home with me, and we could continue to communicate without the work or presence of a therapist. Later I became aware of different sizes or force levels of angels who had different purposes. Then I saw greater beings of light, such as archangels and ascended masters, as I became increasingly schooled in the hierarchy and purposes of our universe.

I watched my clients with growing amazement as I became aware of how the "laboratory of life" was enhancing my own awareness. I was becoming increasingly effective in the classroom and in my duties, which involved the teaching of professionals at criminal justice agencies. My job, I came to realize, was about much more than imparting knowledge about criminal justice. It was to help my students explore their own feelings and their fears. I'd always had a few students come to me, for example, after a lecture on sexual assault. Often they would admit, usually for the first time, the need for assistance with a personal trauma.

Occasionally a student would come to me asking for help, because the spirit of a deceased loved one was appearing or perhaps attempting to communicate. One young man came to my office to talk about a recent death. The grief resulting from the loss of a loved one had put him behind in my class. As I conducted therapy on him, the departed spirit came to the young man to assure him that the decision to have life support removed had been the correct one, though it had resulted in death and transition. In another session with a different student, a departed spirit brought so much love that I was filled with tears. Another student saw a film about Nazi concentration camps and knew that he had died in one.

My clients were having supernormal experiences leading up to personal spiritual awakenings. Yet little had been written to encourage what I now consider an extension of death and near-death experiences: the vivid remembrance of childhood and past-life experiences, and the visitation by spirit entities. I now realize that every individual has access to higher realms of understanding, which my clients and I had tapped into. This access is limited only by an ignorance of how to proceed or by the fear of appearing foolish. It is my goal with this book to do my part in breaking down the barriers — by helping to remove or lower the resistance of social workers and counselors who cling dogmatically to outmoded, modernist, secular views. My wish is to open their minds, and those of all seekers, to the value and efficacy of spiritual experience, so that it can begin to play a role as an important tool in psychological and emotional healing.

When I began writing this book, it was with the intention that it would be for therapists, that it would give them new techniques and insights they could incorporate into their practices. Then I realized that my efforts should be on behalf of the clients of therapists as well, and all seekers who wish to heal themselves. When Pearl first came to me, for example, she had already been experiencing memories of past lives. The only help she needed was for me to muscle test her to confirm the stress, and to help her understand the pattern these memories displayed. Then I was able to assist her in changing her belief system, so that she was able to create the world she really wanted.

Stressful thoughts weaken our muscles and our body. Once I explained this and showed her how kinesiology worked, Pearl was able to work on the smaller problems herself. Only the most difficult required my attention. As I have often found to be the case, she then became my teacher. During our sessions together I learned the truth about the universe and the purpose of our lives on this earth.

I wrote this book for you — therapist, client or seeker. I wish to share with you the process by which the choices for healing can be made — choices to do with situations you may have set in motion in another time or place or life.

— *Mary Clement*
August 1998

INTRODUCTION

Pearl, one of my patients, has agreed to recount her experience in therapy, so you can understand from her experience how the techniques work that I will cover in this book. The purpose, then, of the narrative that follows is to bring to life the process of kinesiology/results therapy by allowing you to be there with her; and to see and feel through her senses and thoughts. Below, Pearl tells the story of her final visit to my office, just as it took place. Here it is, with only minor editing for clarity:

> I felt anxious as I arrived, I guess because later I was planning to visit the present-day incarnation of Robert, and I wanted our meeting to go well. Following the usual greetings, Dr. Clement instructed me to get my entire brain limbered up and working by using the cross-crawl. This is a simple exercise: Touch the left hand to the right knee, and the right hand to the left, while humming and moving my eyes to the left, right, up and down.
>
> Dr. Clement took my thumb and forefinger in her two hands as she had done so many times. She said she could feel my stress. She asked my body at what other age there had been a situation that had caused similar stress.
>
> "Hold your fingers ," she said. "Don't let me pull apart. Okay. Age one to five?"
>
> "Age six to ten?"
>
> This continued until we reached the age of 26. Though I held my fingers as tightly as possible, they came apart.
>
> She asked if the event involved a male. My fingers parted again.
>
> "Age 26. Stress. Male," she said.

The entire scene flashed in my mind. I was married. My husband, a graduate student in art, was shouting at me, "You should do this! you should do that!"

Should, should, should. And always my responsibility.

Taking my fingers again, she asked if we needed to know more about this situation. My fingers came open.

"Was the event positive?"

My fingers became weak.

Dr. Clement said, "What was positive about that time?"

"I would sit back and watch. I just didn't understand, or believe how angry he was, or how everything could be my fault. I blamed myself for some things but certainly not all of of our problems."

Taking my fingers again, she said, "Stress. Male."

Another scene came to mind. "My husband wanted me to pose in the nude for him so he could do an assignment for a graduate class in photography. If I didn't, he'd have to pay someone. We couldn't afford that. I didn't like the idea, but agreed to do it in the privacy of our home. It was daylight. Our baby was awake, and we took her with us to the empty room in the attic. After he took his pictures, he wanted to have sex with me. I submitted and hoped it would end quickly.

"Several days later, he showed me the proofs of the photos. He said he thought they'd turned out well. So well, some of the other male students wondered if I would pose for them. I was devastated and shouted, 'No!'"

Dr. Clement tested my fingers again. They came open again when she said, "Stress. Female."

"I felt so angry inside," I said. "How dare he show

those nude pictures to others. I felt violated. I was his wife, and he was willing to lend me out."

She continued with my fingers. They came open for positive, and she checked to see if this new positive situation had to do with a male or female. Since my muscles were strong on male, she pulled and my fingers became weak on the word female.

"Positive. Female," she said.

I had to think for a minute. What could possibly be positive? Then it came to me. "One photograph was very nice. The soft light on my body created smooth, attractive lines. It was warm, soothing."

Dr. Clement continued to question me. "Hold your fingers together," she said.

Then she'd ask and pull. Depending on whether my muscles remained weak or strong, she'd say positive or stressful, male or female.

"Stress. Male," she said.

"There was no way to satisfy him sexually. He'd make me go to his school, where he worked in the evenings. He'd want me to dress in something provocative and loose so that I'd be available for him. He felt there was less love for him because of the baby, that I should try harder to please him."

"Stress. Male."

"We had no money. He was going to graduate school and I wasn't working outside the home. It affected the food we ate. Too much sugar. It wasn't good for my mental and emotional well-being. We were living off the money I'd earned from a previous job, and I think that made him feel emasculated. He couldn't rule me with money, so he used sex instead."

"More stress. Male."

"He had an affair. I was now being compared to other women. I began to doubt myself. Something must be wrong with me, I thought. I must not be doing it right. I was wearing kiss-and-make-up nighties, reading porno material for advice. My job was to please him no matter how much he deprived me of my spirit. His demands were unreasonable. I remember him wanting intercourse in strange places. One time it was in the middle of this farmer's cornfield. My greatest fear was that a combine or tractor would come down this field, and I wouldn't be able to get away fast enough. What love I'd had for him died. His demands destroyed our intimacy. Then it moved to oral and anal sex."

"Stress. Female."

"The oral sex was choking, uncomfortable."

Dr. Clement softly asked, "Could this have been rape?"

The thought struck me hard. "Yes, rape. He forced me. He was destroying my soul."

"More stress. Female."

"He bought a huge oak bench at an auction for my anniversary. It would never be valuable, but I had to refinish it. He couldn't sell his sculptures, his paintings or photographs. Sometime his ceramics would sell, but it wasn't a good living. He lost focus, lived in a fantasy world."

"More stress."

"He was going to school. I felt obligated to him. He even wanted sex in his studio. I felt like an object. I'd bring the baby with me. It was awful. We were supposed to be a family."

"Stress. Male."

"He didn't get along with his teachers. He lacked friends and support. He had a girlfriend at school. I sensed that he told her his troubles and that she believed him. I think she probably blamed me for not being a good wife, for not understanding him."

"That's enough from age 26," Dr. Clement said. "Now I want you to relax and go back in time."

Sometimes when Dr. Clement told me to relax and go back, I had difficulty because I'd see or feel two different scenes. "I see myself as a maiden. I see a castle, and a church. A high stone wall. Is this the time we're looking for?"

She checked my muscles. I tried to understand where I was. The wall and the church had vanished. I was a young girl. I felt a man on top of me. I was small. He was big, heavy. Smothering.

"I'm small, about age 8 or 10," I said. "There's a man on top of me. My father — my father from Robert's time."

The truth had surfaced. It was no longer a guess or a feeling of intuition that my father of that time had committed incest with me. It was real. I was reliving it.

"Stress. Male."

"Oh, my God!" The realization came crashing in. "My husband of this life was my father in that one. He had sex with me — oral sex and intercourse."

"Stress. Male."

I concentrated on my breathing to get hold of myself. Several moments passed. "I'm lying on a bed and feel this huge man on top of me. He's punishing me. I took away his wife. He says I'm to blame. He feels he has a right to do this. He's doing this to punish me. He is very angry."

"Positive. Female."

"I am protected from others. They don't know what he's doing."

"More positive."

What could be positive about this? "I feel the warmth of his body. He's teaching me about male domination."

"Stress. Female."

"He will not let me see others. I can see myself meeting Robert. I feel his love — something my father never gave me. Robert and I were intimate, but not so much physically. We shared private moments, smiles. We shared our hopes. Our love was sweet, and that frightened my father. I felt wonderful, exuberant, feminine — beautiful and lovely."

"Stress. Male."

"It hurt Robert to the core when he was told he could never marry me." I started to cry and tried to hold back the pain and the remembrance.

"Let it out, Pearl."

"My father denied him our marriage. It broke Robert's heart."

"More stress. Male. Robert."

"Robert didn't want to see me anymore. We talked in code and left messages in books in the library. He felt he was the head of his family, and needed to graduate to help support his mother financially. He chose his mother over me, but he didn't know he could have had us both.

"She was difficult to live with. Then he married

someone else, and she was difficult, too. She and others used Robert's name to make money. His wife got the money, eventually, but she had to wait until his death. Robert's integrity wouldn't permit him to take money without expending effort."

"Stress. Female."

"Seeing someone you love and not being able to love them physically. I can see myself working as a servant for Robert during the Civil War. I'd help him in his quarters. I was near him often, but we never touched or embraced. He wanted to protect my reputation. He wanted to protect me from the other men, so he kept me close by. It was very unusual to have a 'good woman' around the battlefields. He wanted to make sure I was not confused with the prostitutes who worked the camps.

"He also wanted to make sure I would live through the war. He always knew where the battle was going to be, so he could protect me. But we never had a place. No house. No place of our own. We were always moving. Robert got tired, so very tired. There was no rest for him — especially toward the end."

"Stress. Female."

The realization hit me. "I never told him I loved him." I began to cry profusely, the guilt welling up. "I never told him. Never told him.

"After the war it was difficult for us to get together, even though that is all we wanted. He settled in a town in Virginia, and got me a job taking care of someone. In the afternoons he'd ride his horse to come see me. He'd tell the others he was just paying his respects, but the truth was that we saw each other every day. But we had no privacy.

Occasionally, we'd spend a few quiet moments in the garden. I sensed that people felt an old man deserved some love in his life. So they left us alone.

"Then one day, as he walked down the path to my house, he literally fell into my arms. He grabbed his heart. My God, he was having a heart attack! Oh, how I loved him. I couldn't allow him to die at my place! I knew I must get him to the city as quickly as possible — to his house, to a doctor. I hitched a horse to a wagon. It wasn't easy. It had been a long time. I can see myself putting him in the wagon, and driving that wagon with his horse hitched behind it as fast as I could. I headed into town, praying he'd hold on."

"More stress. Female."

"I had to leave him. The person I worked for needed me in the mornings and evenings, so I couldn't be with Robert all the time. I can see myself in his bedroom. I wanted to stay. I sensed that his wife wanted him to die. I just wanted to hold him, but there were people around, so many people. It was difficult to talk with him and tell him what I wanted to say . . .

"I see myself coming back to him one day. Robert had gone into a coma."

"More stress."

"Robert wants to die now. He's out of the coma. He says he's had an experience. Today we'd call it a near-death experience. I'm at his bedside. He's telling me how nice it is on the other side, and that the work we don't complete in this life can be finished in a different way . . .

"He was good, and he was honest. He told me he didn't like the fact that he was in love with me, and married to someone else. He felt that wasn't honest. Yet the near-death experience brought him peace and understanding. He was reassured by some heavenly being that there was purpose in death for his men. He had not been to blame for their deaths or the war. His defeat in battle had not been punishment for loving me. He no longer had to take the blame."

I paused. Dr. Clement asked if we were finished with that event. My fingers went weak, meaning no.

"More about the near-death experience,"she said.

Experiencing those memories was painful, but I knew that if I didn't continue, I'd never banish my demons. So I relaxed, and let it come.

"He saw the white light," I said. "He'd been there, at the edge, ready to enter, and instead he returned. The room had been crowded with family members and friends, but Robert shared with me alone what he had seen and experienced. He loved me. He wanted to be with me.

"There was more Robert wanted to do in life, but he had been reassured that his death was not the end. His work would be finished in another way, in another time. But even so, he came back. Only after telling me, explaining to me, did he feel comfortable in leaving."

Dr. Clement said, "Have we had enough about this life? Hold your fingers." She pulled. They held together, an affirmative response.

She asked if there were any other ages we needed to explore. Then my fingers went weak. So she again used my fingers to determine which.

"0-5, 6-10, 11-20, 21-30, 31-40 . . . "

When she got to age 41, my fingers became weak. She

tested for positive or stressful, male or female.

"Age 41. Positive. Male," she said.

The image came quickly. "I see the minister of my church. He respects me. The minister has a good relationship with his wife. She's a strong woman. He has a good sense of humor. When other women have difficulty in their lives, he refers them to me for help."

"Hold your fingers," Dr. Clement said. "Do we need more about this time?"

My fingers held. We were through with all this emotional release.

Dr. Clement then asked questions about the next step to take. My fingers became weak when she asked about belief systems.

"We are now ready to address belief systems," she said.

She went through her notes to uncover subconscious, erroneous beliefs that needed to be corrected. For example, because I'd called the the minister's wife a "strong woman," she felt that I didn't believe a man could love a strong woman. Also from this session, she felt that I did not believe that husbands and wives could be intimate. To verify this, Dr. Clement asked me to repeat this phrase: "Men can love strong women," as she muscle-tested me.

My fingers went weak.

She said that to attract a man who can love a strong woman, I must believe in my heart that it is possible.

A few other destructive ideas buried in my mind that she helped me discover included a belief that the role of a wife is to be a servant to her husband; that my female aspect feels a need to have power taken from it; that my male aspect feels compelled to break the bond of intimacy; that my female aspect feels unsafe with my male aspect.

In order to banish these misconceptions and to replace them with their opposites, in past sessions Dr. Clement had me make a movie of the old, stressful events. I would view them over and over, as I moved away from them. This allowed me to gain perspective on the events and, finally, to release them. But this time her muscle testing indicated that the use of my neurovascular points would produce the best results. Holding these points, which are located on a person's forehead just above the eyes, helps produce an alpha wave. This causes the individual to process information at a deep level. How long the neurovascular points need to be held for the new belief to sink in is determined by muscle testing.

During our session using this form of meditation and the holding of neurovascular points, Dr. Clement would say the new, desired belief, and I'd repeat it. She would hold my neurovascular points for the length of time which had been indicated.

At the end of our session I was able to keep my fingers together when she repeated the new belief. This indicated that I'd accepted it at the subconscious and conscious levels.

Afterwards I could see the patterns and trace my own reactions to them. For example, I'd been a victim of my father in Robert's time. Because of this, I believed that men would continue to hurt and abuse me sexually. That's why I'd attracted a man who thought a woman should be controlled using sex. The two men — my father in Robert's time and my husband in this time — were identical in my mind. Whether or not the individuals in fact were the same wasn't the real issue. What was important was that the old beliefs continued to attract similar situations and circumstances. To be whole, I needed to get rid of that belief.

Now I understood my relationship with my husband at the age of 26. Divorcing him had been extremely difficult, but it had been the right thing to do. Divorce had released both of us , and enabled us each the opportunity to heal.

With all that baggage holding me in check, no wonder I'd never told Robert that I loved him. Now, for the first time, I saw the pain from Robert's point of view. It'd been so great that he'd withdrawn from my presence. He hadn't been angry with me, only attempting to cope. And he'd had to wait all those years before he could reconnect. How much simpler it would be, I realized, if we would make amends and attempt to correct our wrongs while we are alive. Otherwise, our mistakes follow us through the ages and encumber us.

This is what I learned: Love is most important. It was love that called me into remembering. My love had sent Robert from this earth in another time and space. Love can sustain us until we return to the one great source of Eternal Love. The veil that separates the physical and spiritual worlds is thin. When we come to this earth, the veil of forgetfulness is drawn over our eyes. It is love that lifts the veil. It is love that causes our hearts to swell, our eyes to moisten, our spirits to expand. Love creates more love to fill the void of darkness and pain.

We are never really alone. Whether on this side or the

other side, someone loves us.

When two people are married but not in love, the energy between them is not the kind that heals, nourishes or brings prosperity. When people marry for social standing or wealth, it hurts them. It was not by accident that Robert died of a heart condition. We can all teach ourselves this lesson the hard way, as Robert did. Or we can learn what Robert now knows: Love of the heart is most important in life. And death.

— *Pearl*

Then you will know the truth,
and the truth will set you free.

—John 8:32

CHAPTER ONE
DESIRE

The process of overcoming what separates you from inner harmony begins in the heart, with desire. When using healing techniques called kinesiology/results therapy with clients, I am often amazed at how the mind fools us. Because we believe something in our heads, we also assume that we believe it in our hearts. And that's not always true.

I use muscle testing techniques on clients to determine the belief system that exists in their heart of hearts. Invariably, they're surprised to find their arms or fingers can't withstand the pressure I put on them when analyzing a characteristic they think is a core value, but which they really don't believe deep down.

The client will say, "Yes, I believe in treating people fairly, and I think I'm fairly treated." The client makes such statements to be socially accepted, but her life experiences may undermine such a belief. A client may consciously believe she is being fairly treated, yet feel in her heart that she is not.

Inner conflict and disharmony

During muscle testing I have found that some clients, for example, can hold strong for the belief, "I want to be well," yet simultaneously hold strong for the belief, "I want to be sick." Thus, both statements can be said to be true. Unless something is done to weaken the belief in sickness, the individual will continue to experience illness in spite of her seemingly contradictory belief in wellness.

Some self–help books promote the idea that one merely has to think good thoughts in order to be well. It is true that good thoughts are nourishment to the soul. Yet the reality is that wellness begins in the heart. The first step, therefore, in helping people achieve harmony within and heal, is teaching them to get in touch with themselves in order to determine what they truly want in their heart of hearts.

Recently, research into stress reduction and the role that the heart plays in stress has revealed that communication between the heart and the brain begins in the HEART, not the brain. An early study by HeartMath (IHM), founded in 1990 by Dr. Lew Children, measures the effect of positive and negative emotions on levels of IgA (S–IgA) in the saliva of patients. You see, IgA is an integral part of the immune system. The results show that patients who feel appreciation, care and compassion toward themselves have much higher levels on average. It follows, therefore, that these "feelings of the heart" have a tremendous impact on our ability to ward off disease.

Another HeartMath study finds that heart rate variability is an indicator of mental and emotional states. HRV measures the balance between the sympathetic nervous system that speeds up the heart and the parasympathetic nervous system that slows down the heart. Using an electrocardiogram (ECG), researchers report dramatic differences between the frequencies radiated by the heart throughout the entire body when someone was feeling frustrated, compared to periods when they felt appreciated. The study also revealed that the heart's electrical system is 40–60 times stronger than that of the brain. The electrical frequencies by the heart are so strong that they can be measured anywhere in the body.

The implication of this is that the heart's messages are so strong that they affect every atom and cell of our being. In other words, these vibrations affect our very soul. The goal of kinesiology/results therapy, therefore, is to create an environment in which the client is able to achieve harmony and order, or coherence, in the body's electrical system. Experiences of anger, frustration, anxiety or stress create incoherence in the heart's frequencies. These negative frequencies then send what I call "earthquakes" throughout the entire body, disrupting all kinds of normal functions. On the other hand, when people experience a deep sense of love, care or appreciation, their heart frequencies become coherent and ordered, and the entire body experiences peace and healing.

The bottom line is, the process of healing must begin in the heart. This is more than mere words. Ask any alcoholic or chain smoker if they have a desire to change. Most will say they do. But it isn't as easy as some people make it out to be.

Become aware of two selves within

Napoleon Hill is the one who put his finger on the reason. In the early part of this century, he was employed by Andrew Carnegie to discover what made some people successful, and others not. Hill might have been compared to Abraham Maslow or Stephen Covey today. He devoted his study to the habits that help people self–actualize, and he wrote about his findings.

Hill wrote *Think and Grow Rich* and other best-selling self-improvement books. His work tells how to increase all riches, and not just monetary wealth. His topics deal with the absoluteness of purpose, love, the master mind, applied faith, the law of cosmic habit-force and self-discipline.

In *The Master—Key to Riches,* Hill explains that all of us have two selves. Within each person dwell two distinct personae, and the physical self is simply the house for these two selves. One self is positive and wants sound health, love, friendship and personal achievement. The other self, the negative self, thinks, moves and lives in an atmosphere of self–doubt, fear, self–criticism, judgment and condemnation. The negative self can generate a constant dialog about fear, poverty and concern about ill health. The negative self expects failure, and is seldom disappointed.

Some call this negative self the "not–self." Zig Ziegler calls it "stinking thinking." But this negative self is more than just thoughts. Saint Paul called this negative self "the dweller on the threshold," the force that makes people do the things they wish they wouldn't. It prevents them from doing what they know is right.

Thoughts are things

In the preface to this book we touched briefly on the concept of a Collective Unconscious, or Universal Mind. Each of us is part of and connected to this through our individual subconscious mind. It helps me understand the implications by thinking of this Collective Unconscious as an actual place, not just as an abstraction. It is the fourth dimension, the location of the spirit world. All thought exists here. We can tune into particular thoughts, positive or negative, and in effect channel them into our lives. As the psychic Edgar Cayce said, "Thoughts are things." They do not originate with us. They aren't something we have, or process. Thoughts come to us from the fourth dimension. We have the ability to accept them — welcome them into our lives. Or to reject them.

The significance of this is reflected in another saying that Cayce is famous for. He was fond of quoting Proverbs 27:3, "As a man thinketh, so is he." In other words, our lives are reflections of our thoughts. Positive thoughts result in positive outcomes. Negative thoughts manifest as negative circumstances.

Have you ever noticed that it's the people who talk about real or imagined health problems, those who worry most about getting sick, who most often have physical ailments?

Of course, there are people who really don't want to heal. In the vocabulary of Transactional Analysis (TA), a psychotherapy developed by Dr. Eric Berne, some people play games such as, "Ain't it awful?" Their tales of woe make soap operas seem like comedies. They appear to enjoy having bigger problems and more difficulties than the next guy. And the truth is, these individuals indeed usually do have an inordinate amount of trouble in their lives.

When I make suggestions to them in therapy, they often respond, "Oh, no! Not me, Dr. Clement. I don't *want* these problems. But, you know, the most horrible thing happened to me the other day. Did I tell you? You're not going to believe this, but...."

You get the picture. They seem to relish their pain. To savor it. And, until they change their thinking, until they have the desire deep down to do so, it will continue.

Clear out the negative

Perhaps you see a little of yourself in what I've just described. If you've become overloaded in your life, if you're sick of wallowing in the mud and want, instead, to soar among the clouds, now's the time to begin your transformation. Use the following exercise of the "two columns" to help you understand the power this book will place at your disposal. Take a few minutes to identify these two parts of your being — the negative and the positive. In one column, called the True–Highest–Being–Self, list all the qualities in you that make you glad to be alive. In the second, called the Little–Negative–Untrue–Self column, identify times and example of when qualities such as greed, pride or lust became so important that others' feelings and needs were trampled.

Hill explains that the negative personality that dwells within can become like a radio receiver or a magnet, attracting negative experiences to you. It can become a beacon, guiding negativity to you that you would never choose if you were in your right heart. On the other hand, when the positive personality that lives inside is in control, it attracts a higher energy. It attracts goodness to you, and positive thoughts, and a feeling of hope that translates into an "I can do it" attitude. Hill calls the values of "sound health, love, hope, faith, peace of mind and happiness, the values of life for which you and all other normal persons are searching."

Understand that the negative self has the power to sabotage your deepest desires, and you will be better equipped to make constructive choices. Denying the existence of the negative self allows it to live undercover in the shadows of your mind. Acknowledge its existence. Bring it out of the closet, and into the light. This will enable you to put it in its rightful place, so that you can move on. As Hill explains, the negative self is always with you, but it need not always be in control. Like switching TV stations with a remote control, you can switch to another channel. You can connect with your own positive self, and this will attract other positive selves. This can help to create a more positive consciousness for our entire society.

A Zen Buddhist took a wayward student to a river, where he held the young man's head under water for a few seconds. The young man came up gasping for air. Again, the Master held his head under the water, and brought it to the surface for air. The third time, when the youth was really gasping, the Master said that he hoped the youth would desire to learn as much as he was desiring not to breathe water. We need that kind of desire to truly change.

In *The Seven Spiritual Laws of Success,* Deepak Chopra reminds us that this desire to change must come from the heart. But not the kind of heart that is mushy and sentimental. Rather, he says:

> *The heart is intuitive; it's holistic, it's contextual, it's relational. It doesn't have a win-lose orientation. It taps into the cosmic computer -- the field of pure potentiality, pure knowledge, and infinite organizing power -- and takes everything into account. At times it may not even seem rational, but the heart has a computing ability that is far more accurate and far more precise than anything within the limits of rational thought. (p. 44)*

The desire we are talking about comes from a heart with deep devotion.

The following story from Sogyal Rinpoche in *The Tibetan Book of Living and Dying* (p. 93–94) tells it best:

> *At the time of Buddha, there lived an old beggar woman called "Relying on Joy." She used to watch the kings, princes, and people making offerings to Buddha and his disciples, and there was nothing she would have liked more than to be able to do the same. So she went out begging, but at the end of a whole day all she had was one small coin. She took it to the oil merchant to try to buy some oil. He told her that she could not possibly buy anything with so little. But when he heard that she wanted it to make an offering to Buddha, he took pity on her and gave her the oil she wanted. She took it to the monastery, where she lit a lamp. She placed it before Buddha, and made this wish:*

"I have nothing to offer but this tiny lamp. But through this offering, in the future may I be blessed with the lamp of wisdom. May I free all beings from their darkness. May I purify all their obscurations, and lead them to enlightenment."

That night the oil in all the other lamps went out. But the beggar woman's lamp was still burning at dawn, when Buddha's disciple Maudgalyayana come to collect all the lamps. When he saw that one was still alight, full of oil and with a new wick, he thought, "There's no reason why this lamp should still be burning in the daytime," and he tried to blow it out. But it kept on burning. He tried to snuff it out with his fingers, but it stayed alight. He tried to smother it with his robe, but still it burned on. The Buddha had been watching all along, and said, "Maudgalyayana, do you want to put out that lamp? You cannot. You could not even move it, let alone put it out. If you were to pour the water from all the oceans over this lamp, it still wouldn't go out. The water in all the rivers and lakes of the world could not extinguish it. Why not? Because this lamp was offered with devotion, and with purity of heart and mind. And that motivation has made it of tremendous benefit."

When Buddha had said this, the beggar woman approached him, and he made a prophecy that in the future she would become a perfect Buddha, called "Light of the Lamp."

When I talk about desire, I'm talking about motivation that comes from the heart — the true, positive self that exists deep down under the facade. I'm not referring to the kind of desire that wants something to feed an addiction, or some other temporal craving such as a bigger house, a newer car or membership in the country club. The desire I speak of transcends time and space.

You have a purpose

I believe that each of us was born with a special gift, talent or combination of talents that no one else possesses in precisely the same way. Our destiny is to put those talents or that gift to work in a way, or ways, that will benefit others. Once we do, we will know true joy. Whether or not we now realize it, this is our deep and unwavering desire. We will come to understand this consciously if we can get in touch and communicate with our positive self. Perhaps this will happen through meditation, perhaps from a dream that comes to us while we sleep. Or the techniques that you will learn as you read ahead may be the vehicle you need.

Think about your inner, unselfish desire. Ask yourself what gift you have. What can you do better than anyone? What do you enjoy? How would you like to spend your time and your life? What do you have to give? It may be something as simple and sweet as the song played by the little drummer boy at the birth of Jesus. It may be a discovery that comes from a special talent you have for seeing the underlying logic of a complicated system. Or it could be pleasure others experience because of a talent you have for putting together just the right combination of spices and ingredients to create a special meal or dish. Perhaps you have a penchant for order that you can use to bring order into the lives of others. Whatever it is, believe me, it is there under the surface, waiting for you to discover. Once you find and begin using it, you will know that you are now "on purpose," and that by following this purpose you will help others, and you will help yourself. This is your deepest desire manifesting in the way that is intended.

Move now to the next step in healing, first by asking, and eventually by finding and cultivating a desire of the heart. In the Brihadaranyaka Upanishad IV.4.5 it is said like this:

You are what your deep, driving desire is.
As your desire is, so is your will.
As your will is, so is your deed.
As your deed is, so is your destiny.

May you have at your core a desire so in tune with your soul's destiny that your possession of it becomes a call to the universe that compels an answer from the heavenly hosts.

CHAPTER TWO
TAKE RESPONSIBILITY FOR YOUR CURRENT SITUATION AND YOUR FUTURE

Regardless of what you may think, or would like to believe, you are not at the mercy of forces that are outside yourself or beyond your control. The truth is, you are where you are today because of the decisions you have made and the actions you have taken over the course of your life up to this moment. Taking responsibility means accepting the reality and inevitability of the law of "cause and effect." Some call this the law of the harvest — what you send out comes back to you. Others call it karma. The word "karma" means action — the power latent within actions, and the results that our actions bring.

The law of karma

In many parenting programs today, parents are taught to use natural consequences as a way to help children understand that what happens is a result of their choices, and that they have control over their choices. A time comes when the parent stops telling the child to wear his mittens when he goes outside to play in cold weather. Instead, the parent lets the child dress himself. If the child doesn't want to put on mittens, the parent allows him to go outside anyway. Eventually, the child will come running inside with cold hands, asking for the mittens. The law of karma, the natural and inevitable outcome of what we do, has now been demonstrated to the child.

Some say this law operates on a cosmic scale. No action or thought, whether good or bad, can be released without having an effect. Jesus, for example, often said that a man, like a tree or a vine, should be judged by his "fruit." By this Jesus meant the circumstances of a man's life, which have been brought into reality by his thoughts and his actions. This natural law operates as surely and consistently as any other. Once we become conscious of this, we can begin to exercise control that will shape our personal environment and what we experience.

Once I worked with a woman whose husband was an alcoholic. She hoped he would change. Yet, without realizing it, she repeatedly took responsibility for him. She told me how he came home so drunk one night that he drove his car onto the lawn, rather than into the garage. He then came inside and vomited on the living room rug. Before he woke up the next morning, she had cleaned up the vomit and moved the car.

This client said she wanted desperately for her husband to change. She prayed for him to become more responsible. She was beside herself with anxiety, and was in the process of debating with herself whether it would be best for her and her children if she divorced him.

She asked my advice. I asked her, "Would you permit a total stranger to walk into your home and vomit on your living room rug?"

"Oh, no," she replied. "I'd never permit that."

"Then why do you permit your husband?"

With a few simple questions I helped her see that her co-dependency was robbing him of the opportunity to learn from his actions. I suggested that the next time he left the car in the front yard, she let it stay there. I looked into her eyes, poured love from my heart and said, "Let him clean up his own messes. It's the only way he'll ever learn."

She followed my advice. She told me later that their relationship became more difficult before it got better. But she persevered in her hands-off policy, and this allowed him to learn from the choices he made. As a result, she found she had more time to concentrate on herself and her own needs. In the end the couple remained married, and both became better people, although it indeed was rocky for a time.

Take responsibility

In my experience working with women in prison and in correctional halfway houses, I have come to the realization that many, if not all, are there because they don't take responsibility for themselves. Therapy almost always reveals that this characteristic became established in them when they were very young. It could have stemmed from having parents who didn't give them enough love, and it also could have come from those who may almost literally have smothered them with it.

Jane, age 40, was an inmate at the Virginia Correctional Center for Women. In therapy it became clear that she viewed beliefs as though they were set in stone, and clung to them with usual tenacity. As a child she had been given up for adoption. On the one hand, this made her feel at the subconscious level that she had been abandoned. On the other hand, she felt guilty because she was materially better off than she would have been had she remained with her birth parents.

By the age of 28, Jane was a single parent with two children. She received no financial assistance from the children's fathers. She worked two jobs, which was necessary for her to support herself and the children, but felt guilty she wasn't able to be with them more. Her life history displayed a pattern of unhealthy relationships with men who couldn't, or wouldn't, support or assist her. She found relationships that might have been supportive to be boring, and she consistently terminated these positive relationships. She believed herself to be independent. In reality she had a deep fear of being or becoming dependent, thus opening herself to the possibility of the pain of abandonment, or the guilt of having more than she felt that she deserved. Hers was a no-win situation. She partied and drank heavily, because she thought it made her happy. Of course, it didn't.

Guided visualization

One therapeutic technique successfully used in Jane's case was guided visualization. In these sessions she identified what she needed to do to revamp patterns, perceptions, beliefs and attitudes in order to change her life. Jane saw opportunities that had presented themselves in the past that she hadn't taken advantage of. She saw that she had a deep-seated belief that she didn't fit, which caused her to isolate herself. She realized, for the first time, that for the most part she had focused on her negative inner self, rather than on the positive.

During one visualization exercise, as she moved her eyes up and to the center, Jane realized that her family of origin had put her up for adoption for her own good. Her guilt at having had more opportunities than her biological family could have provided her had kept her from being grateful for the sacrifice that they had made. By going back and recognizing the guilt she had felt, and the pain she had lived with, Jane was able to heal this wound and replace her old beliefs with new ones. She was able to arrive at a deeper understanding, and to know that it was possible to take responsibility for her own happiness. And to allow others to take responsibility for theirs.

Learn to trust

Jane's therapist was able to teach her about healthy relationships by having her use their patient-client relationship as a model. Jane came to see that communication, respect and consideration are integral to a good relationship. With her therapist's support she recalled a time in her life when she had handled things well. It was a time when she had felt loved, needed and wanted. It was a time when people were there for her. She also realized that when she had first left her husband, she had been able to handle life alone, and hadn't needed to ask for help. It was only later that she got off the track and allowed herself to become a victim of drugs and despair.

Jane had been resistant to therapy initially. The kinesiology/ results technique, which was described in the Preface and will be dealt with in more detail in upcoming chapters, helped the therapist to quickly pinpoint Jane's emotional stumbling blocks. The guided visualization allowed her to overcome those blocks more rapidly than might otherwise have been the case. At the end of the five months, Jane openly admitted how improved her outlook had become, and that she now felt more in control of her destiny. Jane no longer felt disgruntled and expressed instead an appreciation for being a part of the program. She was well on the way to recovery.

Identify conditioned behavior

What we now know is that children learn autonomy and self–control between the ages of 18 months and three years. Parents' behavior at this stage of development may teach the child that expressing independence causes suffering to others. For example, if an insecure mother has an emotional need for the child to remain dependent, when the child wanders out of the room she might call out, "Don't go into the next room! You might get hurt!" The dutiful child comes back to the mother's lap but ultimately pays the price for her mother's fears. The child's inner drive for autonomy is denied, and as an adult she may now fear that she will be forever trapped in a symbiotic union of engulfment. According to Harville Hendrix, author of *Getting the Love You Want: A Guide for Couples,* these stifled children often become what he calls "isolators" as adults. These are people who unconsciously push others away in order to gain freedom.

Their opposites, whom they attract, he calls "fusers." They were emotionally abandoned as children; their caretakers were not equipped to handle anyone's needs except their own. Fusers want to "do things together." They crave physical affection and reassurance, and often stay in constant contact with loved ones. An isolator and a fuser together creates a formula for co–dependency.

The codependent person is more than a co–alcoholic, or enabler or one who attracts and mates with an alcoholic. The codependent individual has been conditioned to feel responsible for everything and everyone. Yet, she herself feels powerless and unworthy.

Codependency

Codependency is a situation wherein a person meets another's needs while sacrificing her own. It is a major problem in families with alcohol, drugs or other addictions such as sex, gambling and shopping sprees. Many men and women suffer from co-dependency. Interestingly, domestic violence research shows that not only does the woman who is abused by the spouse feel like a victim, but the husband who abuses feels victimized as well. It is, therefore, difficult to successfully treat abusive men, because they do not see themselves as offenders as much as they see themselves as victims. They feel victimized because they could not get others to meet their needs.

The reality is that no one can fill another's needs or lead their life in the right direction for them. A wife may wish desperately for the alcoholic husband to be sober, and she may take action she believes will result in this. Similarly, the husband may wish his overweight wife to be slender, and heckle or cajole her to lose weight. The truth is that the husband or the wife must take responsibility for themselves. It may help each of them to connect with their higher self, to get in touch with the higher wisdom and power that resides within, in order to provide strength and guidance.

As was stated in the last chapter, personal transformation must begin with desire. Directly to the point of this chapter, the transformation can only continue if an individual then takes responsibility. The husband alone can make the decision to take a drink, or leave it. The wife alone can choose to sneak a piece of chocolate cake in the middle of the night, or to roll over and go back to sleep.

One of the reasons codependency exists in families with addiction is because there are no boundaries. It is difficult to separate good from bad, right from wrong. There is a lot of blaming and excusing of behavior. Some get to the spiritual truth of the matter and call this dynamic "karma–dodging."

Make conscious choices

It does no good to deny the truth. We must step back and witness the choices we make. Then, perhaps, we can begin to make conscious decisions. Often it helps to determine if there is an underlying belief system that needs to be addressed, exposed and deposed. Belief systems are very powerful. Often people will do anything to avoid challenging them. This is what psychologists call avoidance, and it can be very costly.

For years I was a patient of traditional psychotherapies but was frustrated by the process. I yearned for more answers. On occasion I'd meet someone and experience a feeling of love, anger or confusion that was too intense to be appropriate for the particular situation. Prayer and meditation gave me insight into how to deal with these situations. But I was still unclear as to why I reacted so strongly. So I sought out a kinesiology/results therapist. I wasn't hypnotized but was relaxed through natural techniques. The therapist would align my body and hold the neurovascular points on my forehead to produce a deep alpha wave, while I explored my memory.

Examine the past for insights

First, I, like Jane, had to heal the injury created by experiences of this lifetime. Slowly, I began to realize that some of my present-day emotional distress had been put in motion before this life. Remembering far back to a past life may seem like a day-dream, because the image of an entirely different place and time appears in the mind's eye. But the experience is quite different, primarily because the emotions evoked are so intense. Unlike the experience of a dream or a daydream, in a visit to a past life you will feel the clothes of yesterday on your body as they felt then. For example, I have felt the buckskins of an Indian maiden against my skin.

Having someone else administer kinesiology/results therapy gave me greater insight into what was happening in my present relationships. In one former life it seemed that I had been an Indian chief. Through this therapy I recognized that one of my present colleagues had been with me in that time. He'd been an Indian brave, and wanted to be chief without first earning respect, or giving it to others. In my mind's eye I saw myself and this Indian brave together in my tepee. I told this impatient brave to wear my headdress, with all its glorious feathers, knowing full well that the power of leadership is not in feathers or other outer signs of status, no matter how magnificent they may be. Wisdom is in the heart. Power comes from inner strength. Love is the true and lasting tie that binds. This recollection into a past life, whether it was literally a past life or a memory from the Collective Unconscious, gave me insight into my present situation. I realized why my actions had been ineffective and was able to adjust accordingly. This knowledge gave insight that enabled me to overcome the problems I had been facing. But it wouldn't have happened if I hadn't first taken responsibility.

Accept responsibility

When we blame others for our problems, taking charge of life is impossible. Instead we abdicate power to others and in so doing, rob ourselves of the possibility of fulfillment and the joy that can result. Until we accept our current situation as our own, until we accept it as the result of past decisions, we will be prisoners of our stubbornness. Like Jane we will not be able to harness the forces of harmony, joy and love until we look at what we have created and understand that it's our own mess that we need to clean up. Only then will we will be able to create a future that we wish for.

Eastern religions and the traditions of my American Indian ancestors hold that human existence is an almost unending cycle of life, death and rebirth. Rather than reach nirvana, or heaven, we return again and again because we are drawn by earthly desires and the need to clear our unpaid karmic debt. In other words, we continue on the wheel of life because we make errors in judgment.

Once we become aware, however, past errors can be mitigated in order to prevent karma from drawing us back to pay our debt, and thereby learn our lesson in another time and place. Even the most serious of crimes, such as taking another's life, can through grace be overcome by a life of service and surrender to Christ consciousness, rather than to selfishness. So, no matter what you have done, regrets can be changed into resolve, and you can move forward. Once you are devoted to change in your heart, and once you take responsibility for what you create, all you need do is ask, and guidance will come to you. "Seek and ye shall find. Ask, and the answer will be given." The Universe will show the way for you to move through life with joy and thanksgiving.

Meditation

Now, leave the entanglements of your mind and your physical conditions, shut out all discordancy and doubt and fear, and rise into the world of light. Turn your face towards the Sun, the warm gentle sunlight. Breathe in this light . . . it is the life of God, the life which will make you whole. You are spirit, perfect in God.

I am perfect as my Father created me perfect. I am divine love . . . I am divine peace.*

*Source: The Still Voice, The White Eagle Publishing Trust, pages 109-110.

"Move into the wound of your most secret fears,
and find the seeds of wisdom that are planted there.
Face what upsets you the most; it is a great teacher."

— Lynn V. Andrews

CHAPTER THREE
COMMUNICATE DIRECTLY WITH THE HIGHER SELF FOR FASTER HEALING

In recent years Western thought and healing methods have been greatly influenced by Eastern religion and medicine. Kinesiology is a new application of Eastern healing in the Western world. The use of kinesiology as a scientific tool was first practiced in the early 1960s by George Goodheart. Goodheart theorized that for every muscle action in the body, there is an opposing action by a corresponding muscle. A working, tight muscle is strong. If tight muscles cause the hand to clench in a fist, then the muscles that unclench the hand are weak. His conclusion was that we should treat weak muscles rather than put salve on the strong ones.

Biofeedback

Just as chiropractors determine which muscles are strong and which are weak to locate the ailments in the body, the emotional therapist can use muscle testing techniques to determine what events are stressful for a client. Stress weakens muscles so that they can be easily pulled apart. Testing muscles to determine emotional strength concerning events or beliefs is called kinesiology/results therapy. It is a form of biofeedback.

Biofeedback through muscle testing kinesiology identifies conscious and unconscious stress within an individual. Like many mind/body control therapies, kinesiology/results therapy identifies underlying motives of behavior. It helps me to picture how this works by thinking of the involuntary mechanisms of the body as offering a direct link to the intelligence of a person's higher self. The higher self of each of us is always present. It knows all, sees all, realizes what's good for us, what's bad and the course of action that will work out best in each situation. But each of us also has an ego, a little self as opposed to the big self, that has its own desires and needs and agenda. The number one objective of the ego is self-preservation. The higher self views the ego as temporal and could care less about it being preserved. It's concerned with the bigger, cosmic picture. As a result, the ego self will do almost anything to drown out what the higher self would have us know. To block communication the ego throws up a lot of what might often be considered inane chatter inside our heads. This chatter has to do with fears and doubts and inhibitions.

Break through denial

Kinesiology/results therapy makes it possible to break through this smokescreen of denial, rationalization and suppression thrown up by the ego, by allowing communication directly with the higher self through the involuntary functioning of the body's nervous system. This is usually done by means of age regression — going back in time to a specific chronological age or experience). The client is told to hold an arm rigid or to hold his fingers together or in some other way to employ the strength of certain muscles. The therapist mentions certain ages while applying pressure to whatever the client is using his muscles to hold. For example, let's say that the client has been asked to hold his fingers together. The therapist gives the fingers a slight tug as questions are asked. When the muscles go weak at the mention of a certain time frame or age, the therapist knows that this is a a time or an age of importance for the patient.

Pinpoint what needs exploration

During kinesiology/results therapy muscles go weak at the mention of a specific time frame that needs exploration. Once the age is identified, the client is asked to recall the period and to talk about it in order to achieve emotional release.

Usually several meaningful ages and experiences are identified in each session, revealing a pattern of incidents or decisions that led to the individual's present situation. At the root of any pattern of behavior is a belief system. Belief systems are by-products of natural experiences. For example, an adult client who was physically abused as a child might have adopted the belief that she cannot trust anyone. She will continue to validate the belief by attracting, and being attracted to, individuals who are untrustworthy. The old belief may actually have helped the individual cope in the past, but it can be detrimental to the client's present and future. Moreover, it can leave the individual feeling unfulfilled, frustrated and stressed.

Reprogram worn-out beliefs

In order to change and correct what may be an unhealthy situation, one must change one's beliefs. Kinesiology can be of further use in replacing old belief systems with new ones through what is called "emotional replacement." Certain exercises help patients accomplish this. An example is the making of an imaginary movie of the stressful event. Another is the holding by the therapist of the neurovascular points of the forehead to produce an alpha wave state. This and other imagery techniques, including meditation, will be discussed later.

Emotional replacement can quickly bring resolution that dispels old traumas. As a client myself, I consistently left kinesiology sessions feeling at peace, and filled with new confidence in my ability to make the right choices. On the other hand, with family therapy it took longer for me to reach a similar level of understanding and confidence.

When a client shares a present concern, I ask the individual's body, through muscle testing, if it would be helpful to go back in time to a specific age to experience the event, or to delve more deeply into it. I then ask the body at what age the significant event occurred: "0-5? 5-10? age 11? 12?" If the client's muscles go weak at age 6, for example, then I know that something either positive or stressful happened at that time. I then say to the client, "What happened when you were six years old?" Often a memory will come to mind when something positive happened in the client's life. It could be something, for example, that may have provided them with stability. Or they may recall that time in order to discover an important truth. At other times a client's muscles may weaken at the mention of an age when something troubling happened.

Let me give you one example. Jim was a student in my crime and delinquency class. He felt alone. He did not, for example, have a steady girlfriend. I could see that some of the women students were interested in him but, apparently, he missed their signals.

Jim came to me for kinesiology/results therapy. He tested strong for his physical well-being, but his fingers were unable to stay together when I asked about emotional distress. After talking about the stress in his life, I led him through age regression. What period in his life, I wanted to know, should we consider in order to understand this pattern? His muscles tested strong through all ages except the period of his birth.

From what he could tell me about that time, we concluded that Jim's mother had been alone in a big hospital when he was born; her husband had been away in the army. Jim thought his mother probably felt abandoned, perhaps as if no one cared. And as Jim came through the birth canal, he'd picked up that feeling, and it had become a part of his belief system. He believed that he was alone.

When I muscle-tested him for the belief, "I am alone," his muscles tested as strong as a rock; I could not pull his fingers apart. Because of that belief, he'd created a life in which he, indeed, was alone and unhappy.

By way of contrast, Jim's muscles did not test strong for beliefs such as, "Happiness is being alive." His muscles also went weak for the belief, "I now recognize, accept and follow the divine plan of my life as it is revealed to me, step by step."

Using one of the techniques in the kinesiology/results therapy system I will describe later, Jim and I made an imaginary movie in his mind. He revisited the feeling of being alone in the nursery and sensing that his mother was alone giving birth. As he moved his eyes down, he replayed the movie but increased its speed and moved away from it. After this exercise he tested strong on the new beliefs, "Happiness is being alive" and "I now recognize, accept and follow the divine plan of my life as it is revealed to me, step by step." He was now equipped to attract situations that would bring happiness and vitality into his life. He left the session uplifted and strengthened. Most gratifying of all, his life changed immediately.

That evening Jim played in a college basketball game. Typically, he played well on the court, but he missed his foul shots more often than not. Something about standing in front of the basket with his team members lined up on either side triggered his sense of being alone, as though his teammates had abandoned him.

That night he was fouled and given three free throws. As Jim took his position, the crowd groaned, "Oh, no." Jim ignored them, picked up the ball and made the first basket. He took the ball again, bounced it several times and let it fly. It sailed through the hoop. The crowd murmured with surprise. Jim took the ball for shot number three. People began to cheer. The coach appeared to cringe. Jim bounced the ball once. He aimed. The ball hurled through the air and swished through the net. The crowd went wild.

The next day I was strolling across the campus when Jim stopped me. "That was the best game I played all season," he said. I asked if he realized that it had been his "test of abandonment."

A study demonstrates results

Perhaps you wonder if Jim was really cured, or whether he might have had an isolated experience that only made it seem so. I had the opportunity to test the effectiveness of kinesiology/results therapy on a group of drug-abusing female offenders at Virginia's Women's Correctional Institution in 1994, when I oversaw a study at that institution's Goochland Therapeutic Community for alcohol and drug addictions. Participants completed a questionnaire of 130 items before and after receiving kinesiology/results therapy. Results were compared on an individual basis and on the group as a whole, in order to determine if there had been shifts in the levels of self-esteem, life satisfaction, the use of alcohol, passive-dependency, dysfunctional attitude and the prevalence of spousal abuse. In addition to the survey by questionnaire, monthly client progress reports were written by social workers managing the unit. This documented changes in ten areas, including anxiety, avoidance, denial, conscious awareness of feelings, anger, openness, self-initiative, setting boundaries, personal responsibility and peace/contentment.

After six months of kinesiology therapy, improvement noted in the areas of anxiety, peace/contentment and self-esteem was significantly higher, statistically, than results commonly achieved with traditional social work techniques. The social workers involved also commented that, in their opinion, the women involved in the private and the group kinesiology/results sessions moved more quickly toward healing than those who were treated by social workers in the traditional manner. In areas such as passive-dependency, dysfunctional attitude and anger, there was no statistically significant difference between kinesiology and traditional psychotherapies. In all cases, then, kinesiology is either at least as effective as or more so than, traditional psychotherapies. (This research is discussed in more detail in an article entitled, "New Treatment for Drug-Abusing Women Offenders in Virginia" in *The Journal of Offender Rehabilitation*, 25 (1/2):61–81, 1997.)

Two noteworthy cases emerged from that research. First was that of Belinda, a 33–year–old African American. She had been sexually abused as a child and had become pregnant while unmarried at age 17. Her father and grandmother both died the same year.

A pattern her entire family displayed was to attempt to resolve anger through violence. Belinda had watched her brother kill another family member. At age 28 she was sent to jail for killing her brother, an act she committed after discovering him molesting her daughter. Needless to say, she was an angry and confused young woman. She went to great lengths to isolate herself from others due to her fear of intimacy.

Through kinesiology/results therapy, she was able to recognize her pattern of using violence to lash out in an attempt to resolve her anger. This in and of itself was a major accomplishment. But, in addition, she took big steps toward healing. Guided visualization exercises helped her learn to begin to cope with her anger and keep her temper in check.

One reason that Belinda was able to make this progress was that she gained insight about herself and her condition that before had been lost to denial. Never, for example, had she viewed her life at the age of 17 as having been stressful. Only when she continued to fail the muscle test and experienced the involuntary weakening of her fingers, did she begin to realize how difficult becoming an unwed mother and the death of her father and her grandmother had been.

The second case is that of Kathy, a 34–year–old Caucasian woman. Kathy had been abandoned many times, beginning when her father left her. She had, in fact, been deserted in every significant relationship she had ever had. She saw herself as unimportant and irrelevant, and believed that she could trust no one. She became involved in the use of hard drugs and was easily drawn into abusive relationships.

Through guided visualization exercises she began to learn what it can mean to love oneself, to respect oneself and to take responsibility for and ownership of one's own life and happiness. Kathy also had something that anyone who wishes to heal must process: the desire, and a willingness to take responsibility for her actions and the condition of her life. She now has been paroled and is in college, drug-free and doing well.

Kinesiology/results therapy helped mitigate the destructive patterns developed early in the lives of these two women by helping them identify what stressful events had occurred at different ages and the erroneous belief systems that had led them into difficulty. More studies need to be done to explore the range of effectiveness of kinesiology/results therapy, but it seems clear that it is useful in identifying and healing stress that stems from past events.

A memory of conception

One reason why kinesiology therapy may be so successful is because it works with the entire brain. It is one of several psychotherapies that help an individual get in touch with what she experienced during the process of birth. This raises a question: Does a fetus have memories? If the child-to-be is a spirit, is the spirit aware of the environment and what is going on in its proximity? Can it hear and understand the voices of its mother and others? Consider the case of Tom.

Tom was a depressed young man. He had a drinking problem. He felt worthless. He came to his second therapy session accompanied by his father. I had a feeling this was going to be a special event.

The father explained that he had been sending Tom to a psychiatrist, because Tom had been thinking of suicide. Yet when Tom had come home from his first session with me, the entire family had noted a change for the better. The father wanted to meet me and to see what I was up to.

As briefly and succinctly as possible, I explained the techniques I used, and that it appeared to me that Tom was operating with only one side of his brain at a given time. In language I would use with a colleague, Tom would be described as homolateral. Unlike most people, Tom's brain had shut off the ability to process information and stimuli simultaneously with both the left and right hemispheres. As a result, Tom's brain needed to be re-patterned in order for him to regain this ability. This was the reason I was teaching him to do what I call a cross-crawl.

Through muscle testing I'd also discovered that Tom was

suffering from emotional stress that needed attention. After Tom talked about present-day stress he'd been experiencing, using the muscle-testing technique, I asked him if this stress might be related to another time.

His finger muscles tested strong for all ages from birth to his present age, indicating that none of these ages needed further exploration. Then a thought came to me. "What about conception?" His fingers came apart as the word "conception" came from my lips.

I asked, "What do you remember about the time you were conceived?"

He began describing it. He said he felt that the night that his future father and mother had been together, they hadn't known he was there, and they weren't expecting him. Furthermore, once he was conceived and they had learned this was the case, it became clear that his parents didn't want him.

I asked the father if he recalled that night. He was shocked. How, he wondered, could his son have such a memory? What was most amazing, though, was that what his son had said was true. He and his wife had just been "fooling around," with no thought or intention of having another child. Later, when his wife said that she was pregnant again, he hadn't believed it at first. They had a baby just a few months old and already had their hands full.

Tom's belief that he was not planned and not wanted made him feel as if his parents were not there for him. In his mind, he was an unwanted child. But in the presence of his father, Tom went back to see this event as a "movie," and was able to view it differently. What happened that day was cathartic for Tom. His feelings were acknowledged. Obviously, his father appreciated them and understood his son's pain.

All of Tom's problems were not overcome in two sessions.

Considerably more work was necessary. But I relate his experience because it indicates that it may be possible for the spirit of a child to hear and record feelings and events before becoming embodied. This is not unlike near-death experiences, when individuals who have been judged clinically dead relate specific information after resuscitation, such as what the doctors said or that someone in the room had on a mismatched pair of socks. Usually, in such a case the individual will say that he felt as if he was floating above his body, and was able to hear and see everything that was going on.

If an out-of-body experience can occur after death, perhaps it can also occur before conception,which leads to what is perhaps an obvious question. Why not even further back?

Recall of a distant past

Consider the case of Judy. Her memory of a past life was not brought about by a historical movie or by a stressful event in her life. It happened in the therapist's office, where she had come with what she thought was a burning, current issue.

Judy had divorced her husband after a short marriage. Subsequently, the ex went to the leaders of their church to petition their support. It appeared he was trying to continue exercising power over her. She knew that what was brewing wasn't healthy, and decided to leave her church.

The therapist asked Judy to recount her first memory. To the surprise of both Judy and the therapist, when she relaxed her mind the image appeared of herself as a beautiful, young woman lying in a barge, floating down the Nile in ancient Egypt. Several attendants accompanied her. Judy noticed her long, flowing hair, how smooth her skin was and how her fingers were long and tapered. She saw that her fingernails and toenails had been painted. No clouds were in the sky. The sun shone bright.

In her present life Judy loved the sun. She thought, "So this is why, when I am sunbathing, I sometimes think I may have been a sun worshiper in Egypt in another life."

As she floated along the river in her memory, she became aware that she was going to meet a young man. Both were highly respected members of their society. Both were educated. Both were kind, loving individuals whose servants honored them for the just treatment they bestowed.

Judy stepped from the barge and was greeted by the young man. He extended his hand. She placed hers on his, and off they went to a public park to become acquainted. The servants on the barge and the dock smiled, as if to say, "What a perfect couple."

Judy's memory of herself was that she was shy and quiet. The young man had a similar personality. After a time they discovered the love within and between them. As time passed, they grew closer and closer.

One day the earth shook. The buildings trembled. Rocks fell and people scattered. Judy heard the cries of children. At first she thought it was a volcano. Then she realized it was an earthquake. She rushed to find her beloved. People were sprawled around, dead, injured, hungry and thirsty. She pushed at rocks and dug with her hands to find him. But he was gone.

That day something within her died. She mourned, but continued living and serving her people.

Apparently, she had been a powerful person. After the earthquake it was necessary for her to make decisions without the counsel of those with whom she had previously shared responsibility. People would come and attempt to persuade her to accept their point of view. In some cases they planted false ideas in her. Finally the court jester told her what was really going on. He was able to cut through the deceit with a sense of humor that amused her.

Time went on. Her power grew. Yet she always longed for and wondered about her beloved. To make matters worse, she was told that because he had not been buried by the priest in a tomb, his body and soul were lost forever.

Unable to accept this, she began to ask questions of the religious leaders who did the embalming and conducted rituals. They had great power and her questioning of them threatened their authority, so they decided to kill her. In her mind's eye she saw them sneak up behind and stab her in the back.

After her death she left the earth's realm and was reunited with her beloved. They were together again in spirit, but only temporarily. Men in white robes came for her beloved. Women in white robes came for her. In yet another realm she went before a board of wise people and was told that she had accomplished all that she had been sent to do in that embodiment. She was grateful for their reassurance, but wanted to know about her beloved and when, if ever, they would be together.

The wise men and women huddled and discussed this as she waited. One of the holy persons, acting as spokesman, announced that she and her beloved could indeed be together again in another time and place.

The lessons learned

Judy found the memory that unfolded in that therapy session, if it really was a memory, to be helpful and comforting. It explained a number of things about her life. It accounted for her fondness for sunshine, her affinity for Egyptian cotton clothing and bed sheets. She also was able to identify people in her life today. For example, the court jester was her son today, with the ability to cut through deceit with humor. One of the men in the group of priests that had killed her appeared to be one of her co–workers. In this life he only figuratively stabbed people in the back. Even more interesting was that one of the men who'd killed her in the past life was her father, who now was working off the karma he'd created. This was being accomplished by bringing her into the world and giving her the gift of life, and by continuing to give her his support. Judy's appreciation and love for her father became stronger as a result, even though like many children she wished some things about her childhood had been different. Now when they celebrate her birthday, she believes she actually is celebrating her father's decision to give her a birthday in payment of his debt.

Whether or not Judy actually lived that past life, whether it was a recollection plucked from the Collective Unconscious, or whether it was a dream-like fantasy constructed by her subconscious mind, the experience of that "memory" allowed Judy to understand the circumstances and dynamics of her life today. She was able to see, for example, that when she questioned religious leaders, because of their own doubts and fears some invariably will take offense. Because of this and her ex-husband's petition of them, the elders of her church were probably about to turn on her. As a result, her decision to withdraw had been for the best, though difficult and painful. Her departure made it possible for everyone to avoid unconstructive conflict and heartache, including her.

The young Egyptian, Judy now realized, was a fellow student she'd met while on an exchange program at the University of Beirut in Lebanon. Their relationship had been slow to develop because both had been shy. She recalled feeling hurt that he hadn't asked her to one of the school dances. She'd believed he wanted only to sit on park benches with her. She wanted him to acknowledge their relationship publicly. When the school year ended, they had parted because she had to return to America. At their last meeting he had placed a heart-shaped necklace around her neck.

Not long before Judy had decided to enter therapy, this man had called her. To her joy and amazement, she learned that he was living in the United States. Over the telephone he spoke the words that she now believed she'd been waiting to hear for centuries.

"I love you. Come."

Almost beside herself with expectation, she had run to him. Judy wanted an immediate relationship leading to marriage, but the young man, although he felt she was part of him, too, was already married and had two children. He would not, felt he could not, leave them.

For a time Judy was deeply hurt and confused, and it was at this point that she had come for counseling.

It is said that when one has knowledge of others, one is wise, but when one has knowledge of oneself, one is enlightened. Therapy helped Judy make progress in the second category. She learned what she must undo and complete, and what she must master within. She has since forgiven the young man and herself, and is more open to what may lie ahead. We may not get everything completely right in a particular lifetime, but that should not stop us from giving it our very best shot.

I learned many things from Judy. Most of all, I learned about the depth of passion and the strength of drive it is possible to possess. Our desires can push us into situations before our heads realize what is happening. This is why people buy houses that turn out to be money pits — because their desires outweigh good sense. The kind of desire that feeds addictions and other temporal cravings has been allowed the upper hand, and this can be extremely destructive. If we happen to believe in reincarnation, then we also must believe that it can lead us to create karma that may take many lifetimes to undo.

For example, suppose a married person is suddenly strongly attracted to someone other than his or her spouse. Perhaps this love is actually an old love from another time and place. Perhaps not. Maybe it's basic animal attraction. In either case the potential for trouble weighs heavily. In either case strong self-discipline will be required. Many individuals may be hurt if fantasies and desires such as those inherent in this situation are acted upon.

Taking the long view, that this life is not necessarily the only life that will offer the opportunity for two souls to be together, can change for the better the way we regard such a situation. For example, what would have happened if Judy's beloved, having the larger spiritual view, had said to her, "No, not yet. I do not wish to create negative karma with the woman to whom I am presently married. Our marriage is good. Our love may not be passionate, perhaps, but we are supportive of one another and our children. The passionate and longing love that you and I share has been and will continue, but we must wait until later in this life, or perhaps until another, to be together."

He might even have his own memory of an ancient life, fact or fantasy, to explain his situation. "Many centuries ago I had an affair with this woman, and we aborted two children. Now we have been given the opportunity to undo that decision by giving birth and rearing these two children. Once this purpose is completed, then I may be able to be with you again."

Whether it's undoing karma from a past life, not wishing to create it for a future one or simple, common decency and the wish to live up to one's commitments, Judy needed to respect this young man's decision and not to take it personally. Judy's therapist was able to help her see this and understand.

This is not to say, however, that it is always best for married couples to stay together "for the sake of the children" or some other supposedly noble reason. In some cases the correct and logical course is to separate and start anew. This is particularly true of unions that are physically abusive or where mental cruelty exists. The truth is that for many it is much more destructive for children, as well as for the adults, to remain together. People who share their lives need to be mutually supportive. They must put the spiritual growth and development of significant others, as well as offspring, at the top of life's priorities.

Let's have a look at another case.

The case of the four-year-old

A few years ago I was treating a four year-old who had been a victim of sexual abuse while attending day care. She'd been two and a half years old at the time of the incident.

The first clue that something wasn't right came one day when the little girl, Susie, asked if they were going to eat the dog's "poopies" (feces) for dinner. The mother explained to the child that in our society we don't eat that kind of thing. Then the child replied, "We did at day care."

The mother stayed calm, but attempted to find out if anything was really going on.

Small children have difficulty identifying and communicating troubling events. They don't have enough experience to know what's normal and what isn't. They often give information piecemeal, so parents must listen carefully.

Over time Susie gave her mother the impression that ten children had been present when the incident occurred. A man and a woman had also been present. Susie also said that when the lights were turned off, a monkey hurt the children. She also gave the impression that another child pulled her pants down and that the boys urinated on her private area.

As horrible as this may sound, it was only the beginning. The mother met with a great deal of resistance from Child Protective Services as well as the day-care center, and the case never went forward due to the child's age and the lack of physical evidence.

After a while, Susie began to have terrible nightmares. She'd awaken in sweat in the middle of the night. She stuck to her mother like glue.

At the time I was working on a dual degree in social work and law, and was especially interested in helping in the prosecution of sexual child abuse. As part of my social work degree, I had a field placement in Child Protective Services and was becoming knowledgeable about occult crimes. I had also received special training in kinesiology/results therapy, which I thought might be useful with a four year-old child.

The following note written by the mother gives an indication of the situation I was presented with:

> *Friday night, [Susie] was truly frightened to go to bed by herself. So I went to bed with her to help settle her. Again, her stomachaches began. She said something was in her stomach. When she was asked how it got there, she said that it had come through a cut on her leg (there were no cuts at that time), and that it went into her tummy. I asked if it had a name. She said, "Yes, it was Satan." She was very serious. I told her how to command that he leave using the name of Jesus Christ. She did this and then insisted I command him to go, too, because he was trying to get into me. So I did.*
>
> *Last night when she was in the bathtub and seemed to be having a good time, I decided to run downstairs to put some towels in the dryer. She fussed, but I went anyway. Before I finished putting them in, she came down the basement steps*

with her nightgown on. She said she had already washed and dried herself.

If I am quiet for more than two minutes, she starts screaming for me. She acts like a child who was abandoned when she was very young.

On Monday Susie wet herself at nap time. On Tuesday in the late morning, she wet herself for no apparent reason; then she had another accident at nap time. When I asked her why, all she could say was that I hadn't said anything about her accident the day before, as though it had been okay with me.

I gave her no dessert after supper, and told her that she wouldn't have any on Wednesday if there were more accidents. Wednesday's report was good. She was not sassy or uncooperative at school, and no accidents occurred.

On Wednesday morning I got up before Susie did. I was sitting at the dining room table when she came looking for me, wide-eyed and frightened, as if she thought she would not to be able to find me, anywhere.

When I first spoke with Susie, she clung tightly to her mother as we talked about her dreams. She seemed obsessed with "bad monsters" who appeared in her dreams. The bad monsters had "big eyeballs," "huge tails," were as "tall as mommy," had "arms as long as my arms" and they "stepped on [people]." Susie also believed there were monsters in the nightmares "who come back to earth to kill the bad ones."

After about about half an hour I used a technique known as "re-patterning" to help her use both the left and right hemispheres of her brain at the same time. In emotional trauma such as this I have found that it is common for a client to become stuck in either an overly emotional, or overly logical, response to such a stressful situation. Dennison, creator of *Brain Gym*, calls this "switching off."

After re-patterning I began to use muscle testing on the child. Her body indicated that she'd experienced emotional stress at the age of two. At the mention of that age Susie literally climbed into her mother's lap.

Having conducted research on ritualistic abuse, I knew that Satan worshipers sometimes mistreat young children severely. But at this stage Susie didn't want to tell me that she had eaten dog "poopies." By then she'd been taught the significance of this, and was embarrassed about it. These people want a child to believe that she has done something so terribly wrong, so absolutely sinful, that she can never be forgiven. The idea, you see, is to win her over for Satan. Of course, since it is the antithesis of Christianity, the irony is that the Satanists' own line of reasoning would hold that forgiveness is always possible. It can be had for the asking, simply by accepting Satan's opposite, Christ. (According to traditional Church canon, Christ has washed away the sins of His followers, past, present and future, through His sacrifice on the cross.)

By clinging to her mother's bosom, Susie was dealing with her past as best she could. What she needed to know was that she could put this awful episode behind her. It needed to be brought into the open and dispelled. I asked Susie if her mother could tell me the story of what happened. She agreed.

The mother began to tell me what she thought had happened. When the mother was in error, Susie would pull away, insert the correct version and quickly mesh herself back into her mother's neck.

Susie described her nightmares: dragons and slayings of dragons by a mighty warrior with a sword. I was struck by the strong similarity between what was going on in her nightmares and the picture of St. Michael I had on a shelf in my office, and it occurred to me it to give her.

The mother, of course, thought she had the story right. But one detail the child inserted was that the teenage son of the day care worker had taken Susie into another room during nap time, and had hurt her by pulling her pants down and poking her in her private area with a sharp, pointed object.

Employing "movie" therapy

A difficult situation had unfolded in my office. The mother was feeling the impact of her daughter's words for the first time, and the child had so regressed in behavior and withdrawn that I had no idea what might develop. Something was needed to get things moving in a positive direction. So I decided to employ a technique I call a "movie," which is a kind of guided or directed daydream. If effective, the client views the stressful event in the form of a pretend movie while moving the eyes downward and to the right; then downward to the center; then downward to the left. Each time the movie is run, the client is told to speed it up or to run it faster, so that it becomes less personal and less threatening. The eye movement helps the brain access different areas where the memories are stored.

The movie is run again, and the eyes move upward and to the right; upward and to the center; upward and to the left. Each time the eyes shift, the client is told to breathe deeply.

For Susie, when her eyes went up and to the right, she saw a man hurting another man and monsters. When she moved her eyes up and to the center, she pulled away from her mother and sat up. She seemed to be filled with a sense of awe, and reported seeing bright white light. I sensed that for perhaps the first time in a long time she felt safe. Then she moved her eyes to the left, and took a deep breath. She said she saw mountains. Large rocks. I sensed that she had tapped into the strength within her, and she would heal. That everything would be all right.

She moved her eyes to her right, saw stars and said she sensed hugs and kisses coming to her. I, in turn, sensed that my work with her was finished.

She blinked and looked at me. Her behavior had changed miraculously. She no longer appeared to cower. Before, she had tested weak when asked to repeat, "I am confident in all situations." Now, she tested strong. Rather than cling to her mother, she said she wanted to leave.

She got up, leaving her stunned mother behind in the chair. She collected her belongings. She gave off a new aura of confidence. Clearly, she was finished with this session and, for that matter, with therapy.

She was almost out the door when I remembered the picture I'd wanted to give her. I found it, and handed it to her — St. Michael slaying the dragon. I told her that St. Michael protected children and that he would protect her, too. She could put it by her bed.

She looked at the image and her eyes grew wide, as though she'd seen a Christmas tree for the first time with all its lights and decorations.

"Oh, my. But his real sword is so much bigger than that. It reaches to the sky!"

Affirmations/ Belief Statements

I love myself unconditionally.
I love others unconditionally.
Others love me unconditionally.
I am worthy of love.
I forgive myself all perceived wrongs of my past.
I forgive others all perceived wrongs of the past.
Others forgive me of all perceived wrongs of the past.
All my desires are worthy.
I am worthy of all my desires.
I recognize my talents and abilities.
I recognize the talents and abilities of others.
Others recognize my talents and abilities.
I create happy, healthy, loving relationships.
I attract happy, healthy, loving relationships.
I am attracted to happy, healthy, loving relationships.
I am an equal.
I am confident in all situations.

Here (in this experience) all blades of grass,
wood, and stone, all things are One.
When is a man in mere understanding?
When he sees one thing separated from another.
And when is he above mere understanding?
When he sees all in all, then a man stands
above mere understanding.

—Meister Eckhart (1260-1327)

CHAPTER FOUR
YOU AND THE UNIVERSE ARE ONE LIFE

Consider the possibility that everything, including the earth and all its plants and animals, the heavens and all their celestial spheres, is One, a seamless whole, a complete organism unto itself that only appears to be comprised of distinct and separate parts. The idea isn't new. The oneness of creation has been the message of mystics and wise people throughout the ages. The idea is implicit in the ancient Jewish chant, "Hear, Oh Israel, the Lord thy God, the Lord is One." It is present in the modern concept put forth by Carl Jung and other psychologists and thinkers that everyone shares one unconscious mind.

All-Is-One

If we can step back and view things from the largest possible perspective, eventually we will come to accept the idea that creation is one great living organism. It follows that if each human being and, indeed, all things are facets or aspects of a larger organism, then nothing that transpires happens by accident. If nothing happens by accident, we must ask ourselves, is the One Life that we call creation hostile toward any of its parts? Does it wish them ill? Indeed, does it bring misfortune upon them simply for the sadistic pleasure of it?

Would you bring misfortune upon your foot or your hand or your ear simply for the sadistic pleasure of it?

It does not seem likely.

It follows, then, that if things don't go our way it is because the universe is trying to tell us something or teach us something. Yet because there is pain, we sometimes become lost in the pain.

Bad pain, good pain

I recall the time that a neurosurgeon helped me clarify the difference between pain that is healing and pain that is harmful. The surgeon had performed surgery on my neck to remove part of a broken disk that was pinching the nerve that led to my left arm. The pinching was so strong I'd had to carry my left arm with my right. After the surgery I came in to see the doctor and complained that I was still in pain.

The doctor asked, "Is it as bad as before?"

"No," I replied. "But it still hurts, and I'm still forced to carry my left arm."

"What you feel is healing pain, and you will have new growth. If I hadn't operated, you'd never have had new growth, and you'd have continued to feel pain. They're both pain, of course, but the first was harmful. What you feel now is the healing. Think of it in the way you would growing pain."

At last I understood. All was working toward a higher personal growth, though it didn't feel like it at the time. It was then that I began to think of life itself as a classroom. And more importantly, that there was a School Teacher whose job was to teach me by means of the lessons I created to teach myself. Now, after years of observing myself and others in this light, I believe that there's a lesson in everything. When we don't understand this, we become overwhelmed with the pain and start feeling sorry for ourselves, which gets us nowhere.

We ask in anger or outrage, "Why is this happening to me?"

A better approach might be to realize that if we'd been paying attention to the universe, rather than keeping our heads buried in our own egocentric thoughts, perhaps we'd have learned the lesson and gotten the message without having to be hit on the head with a two-by-four.

The story of Mary

Sometimes, a person comes to me with what others might think is an extraordinary circumstance. I view this not so much with awe but as an opportunity to learn. Such was the case of Mary, a professional with a busy schedule who had the opportunity to attend a national conference in the West. Actually, she viewed it more like a chance for a holiday. She'd have some time to herself to relax and watch a few videos she hadn't been able to see at home. One was on King Arthur, the legendary king of ancient England, who'd tried to unite the country with a society of knights who sat as equals at a round table.

While she watched the movie, Mary had deep feelings, more intense than she normally experienced when watching a movie. This particular production had been made a long time ago and didn't benefit from the technology or big-budget pageantry of some of the more recent versions of the story of Camelot. Nevertheless, she said that when it was finished, she felt a tremendous sense of sadness that the king hadn't received the love he'd so deserved. The feeling persisted for days, and Mary found herself reading as much as she could about the legend. She realized that King Arthur, Guinevere and Sir Lancelot probably had been real people. They had tried to establish a higher order of government than had existed up to that point in England. At a time when the rule of despots had been the order of the day, Arthur and his followers had believed that God alone was sovereign, and that under God all were equal. Despite good intentions, however, they failed. It has been said that witchcraft, intrigue and treachery were the root causes.

Mary came to me in a state of melancholy or mild depression that appeared to stem from an erroneous belief system or trauma from an event that may have happened when she'd been a child.

I performed muscle testing to find her age when the belief had been established. Apparently, however, nothing had happened all the way back to her birth. Nothing at conception, either. So I asked, "Past life?"

Her fingers became weak.

Once again, let me interject that it is not my purpose to convince anyone, or even to speculate on whether what a client believes she's experienced actually took place. As previously discussed, it is quite possible that these memories are a sort of metaphor — as are many dreams. They may come about in order to help a client identify what is troubling her. You may prefer to regard them as memories or products of the Collective Unconscious rather than as past lives. What is important are the feelings a client has and the need to bring them to light so that what lies at their root can be determined.

With this in mind I honor an individual's past life "memory" and do not attempt to persuade her that she may in fact be hallucinating. This would be counterproductive. These "memories" can be extremely valuable, as you will see.

One thing that amazes me is the detail with which they often are recalled. One consistent detail has to do with clothing the clients "feel" they're wearing. They may talk about the softness of buckskin or the heaviness of the wool coats of the Civil War era. They usually smell the smells and hear the sounds, though they often relate only a small portion of what is being played out in their minds. I sometimes picture what they experience as a time capsule. The clients go into it to learn a lesson that will help them with their present-day situation.

Other professionals have, by the way, attempted to find proof of past lives told to them in therapy. For example, in the 1970s psychologist Linda Tarazi spent three years checking on one client's story. She was able to identify more than a hundred facts that would not have been known if the client had not lived in sixteenth-century Spain, or at least had access to the memory of someone who did. Dr. Tarazi never was able to prove that an individual with the name her client claimed for that past life, Antonia Ruiz de Prado, actually had lived. Yet, she was able to verify almost every other aspect of the story. "Antonia" accurately gave names and dates that were available only in documents written in Spanish in the town of Cuenca, Spain. The client was from Chicago and had been brought up a Lutheran. She had no Spanish blood, no childhood experience in that area and no educational background to do with Spanish history or the Spanish language.

As I recount Mary's story, I will do so as if it were a single stream of consciousness. In reality a client usually experiences a scene, wonders what it means, and I help her focus on what is stressful for the different characters. This usually transpires over a number of sessions. In some cases the client needs help in seeing the positive elements of the experience. At other times it's negative elements. Often the person represented as a male in the scene is actually a female client's masculine aspect. Likewise, other women may represent feminine aspects, some of which may be suppressed. It is by deciphering and extracting meaning that I can be of greatest assistance. To do so, I simply listen to the memory and determine what was stressful and what was positive. Together, we attempt to pinpoint the belief system or systems that underlie the experiences. This is likely to be what's at the root of the client's problems today. By bringing the beliefs into the open, we can examine them and dispel those that are faulty and destructive. The client is then in a position to create a better future. You see, each individual wishes subconsciously to "prove" the validity of his or her beliefs. We all do so by attracting situations and outcomes that "verify" what we hold to be true.

Let's have a look at Mary's memory:

> "I am a lady-in-waiting for a maiden of aristocratic blood. I'm one of those special women whose job it is to help her plan her activities, to help her dress and manage her personal affairs. I see myself in a very cold castle with walls of stone. I see myself working with her, talking with her and being her confidant.
>
> "Then I meet the king. Oh, I see now. It is King Arthur. He is so tall and handsome. I want to marry him. Instead, he will marry the maiden, and together she and I will go to live with him.
>
> "As time goes on, my love and devotion for the king deepens. The queen suspects my true feelings and introduces me to a knight who proposes marriage. The king thinks it will make me happy to be with this man, so I do get married. . . .
>
> "Alas, the marriage seems to be in name only. . . .
>
> "It doesn't work out. The queen permits me to return to work for her. But now I notice how very much she and Sir Lancelot are attracted to each other. I notice also that the king withdraws and permits their activities by neglect. In time I have the unfortunate experience of finding Lancelot and the queen together. I am torn between my love for and loyalty to the king, and my commitment and devotion to the queen.

"I go to the king and tell him what he knows already in his heart. His queen loves another — his favorite knight. In fact a theme of this court appears to be that people love others' husbands and wives more than they do their own.

"Even if no adultery actually took place between Lancelot and the queen, the king knows that a sexual relationship with her is no longer appropriate or possible. Her heart belongs to another.

"War is coming. The king arranges for the queen to go to stay in a convent, where the sisters will care for her and assure her protection.

"I stay with the king through the battles. He is seriously wounded. Before he dies, he asks me to bury him. Others help me put his body in a boat. But I row it through the misty waters of Avalon, a very special place where the veil separating the physical and mystical worlds is thin.

"I put special weights upon his body and cast him into the sea.

"Then I return to the queen and share the sad news. She forgives me, and permits me to live with her. Soon she becomes sick and wants to die. She tells the sisters she wants to be cremated. I see the shock on the sisters' faces. Since they believe in the eventual resurrection of the body, this is totally opposed to their beliefs.

"Next, I see us outside the gates of the convent. We have been sent on our way.

"I see myself walking in a meadow, leading a horse with a rider who is ill. It is the queen. In the distance I see another rider. My heart sinks. I have no knights to protect me. I have only one horse, and the queen is very sick.

> "I see a second rider who is accompanying the first. I think that my time is up. My heart goes faint.
>
> "As the riders approach, I see their flags. I see their colors. It is Lancelot and his aide.
>
> "My heart is strengthened. I await his arrival. He immediately dismounts and embraces his beloved. Now I am able to see how much they love each other; they are twin flames. I feel sorrow for them. And as she lies in his arms in his embrace, her soul escapes her body. Then, in spirit form, she asks me for permission to use my body so that she can be closer to her lover. This doesn't seem like a good idea to me; nevertheless, I agree and permit it. But it doesn't work, and the plan is abandoned.
>
> "Together, Sir Lancelot, his aide and I ride off to a place where we can prepare the queen's body and cremate it. Then Sir Lancelot has his aide take me to a society of sisters in France. I am safe there but eventually I, too, pass away."

The importance of this session is not the story itself but, rather, the beliefs that it reveals. For example, Mary believed that she had been a servant to both the maiden, who later became queen, as well as to the king. If she continues to hang onto the belief that her role is to be a servant, then it's doubtful she'll ever seek to be president of her company or chair of her department or the head of any club or organization to which she may belong. In her mind only males could be kings. If, however, she were to think of the king as her masculine aspect, and the queen as an aspect of her feminine side that has been suppressed, then she might be in position to picture herself in a leadership role.

A new belief that also would be of benefit is that the queen can be equal to the king. In the time of King Arthur, of course, people did not believe this was possible but in today's society it certainly is.

In Mary's case some of what may seem obvious to you and me was not so obvious to her. Often, grief, sorrow, pain or unexpressed love hinders an individual's ability to see what is truly going on. It would never be a good idea, for example, for her or anyone to permit someone else, even a spirit, to use her body. Subconsciously, she knows this. Doing so would almost inevitably produce feelings of guilt and unworthiness. She has swept this under the "emotional rug," so to speak, but nevertheless, it remains and diminishes her ability to feel good about herself, making it difficult for her to reach her full potential. In order for her to heal, the following affirmations were identified for Mary to concentrate upon in order for them to become incorporated into her belief system:

I no longer permit others to use my body.
My boundaries of self are established.
The boundaries of others are established.
Death cannot separate me from my true love.
The king and the queen and I are equals.
The king and the queen and I are one.
I allow the queen to bond with her true love.
I honor her special relationship.
I no longer carry a sense of failure.
I assign this failure energy to its proper place.
The queen forgives me for following the king.
The king understands and approves.
My love for the king transcends death.
My male aspect is no longer shut off from me.

In Mary's case there were several other beliefs that needed work. What I've given you, however, illustrates the value of examining her past-life "memory." The king is she. The queen is she. The split between the king and queen is really a split within Mary's own being. When she forgives them, in reality she is forgiving herself, thereby permitting a reintegration at a higher level of consciousness.

Scientific support for unity

This brings us back to the thought at the beginning of this chapter: that all creation is one, and we are one with all creation. Modern science seems to have reached a point where it, too, has accepted this concept. According to scientists, the atom now appears to be more like energy, for example, than a thing. Quantum physicists tell us that what happens to an atom here can effect what happens to another halfway across the universe. So no time and space separates atoms, no matter where they may be.

The entire material universe is comprised of atoms. It follows that all *is* one. While we may appear to each other as separate, disconnected beings, each of us is an extension of the whole. I like to think of the whole as the Creator's spirit, and although each soul has its individuality, all souls are of that spirit.

Each soul, then, reflects the whole of creation, and in a sense contains the whole of creation within it. Each is a miniature universe, a model of the larger universe, and is analogous to a drop of water in the ocean. Within a drop are all the ingredients. Within each person is intimate knowledge of all of creation.

Unity is real, even if difficult to believe or grasp. The development in recent years of laser holography has made the concept easier for me to get my mind around. As you know, when you aim a laser beam at a holographic plate, the beam bounces off the plate and projects a three-dimensional picture into space. You can walk around this picture and see the object from all sides. It looks solid and real.

If you were to take that holographic plate and break it into many small pieces, even the smallest would still recreate the entire three-dimensional picture in space. You see, in some mysterious way every tiny piece of the holographic plate contains the entire picture.

A soul might be compared to a piece of the complete holograph that we call creation, or God. Each soul has knowledge of the whole.

Accept all that is within you

For us to become whole, for our souls to have the ability to soar, we must accept all the diverse parts of it. We must bring them all together, even the dark pieces, the shadow selves, and accept them. A part of Mary's masculine aspect and a part of her feminine had become separated. Her "memory" was attempting to tell her this. She was, in fact, Arthur, Guinevere, Lancelot — all of the characters of this memory. But she viewed herself as separate, as the servant, unworthy and therefore unable to obtain the king's love. Even her higher female aspect, Guinevere, was forever separated from her true love, Lancelot. Mary needed to bring all these pieces back together into a unified whole. She literally needed to "re-member" her soul. Once this was accomplished, she was in position to soar. She then could be anything she could imagine herself to be. This realization is what awaits you as well. You simply need to accept it.

The actual process of therapy such as Mary's takes a number of sessions. It doesn't happen in just one, as this condensed example might lead you to believe. Like anything worthwhile, time is required to progress from first step to final resolution. As Mary's fractured psyche healed, additional information surfaced.

Each time this happened, we were able to ask, "Why is this happening now? What is the significance?"

It began with feelings of deep sorrow that lasted several days after seeing an old movie. This triggered something in her, and she acted on it because she was aware that there are no accidents. By asking why, she accepted the Universe's offer to teach her and, ultimately, to heal her. Had she waited, had she dismissed her feelings, she might have lost a golden opportunity. She might even have been pulled into another situation, a Camelot of today, so to speak, that would have resulted in the pain that she instead "recalled" in therapy. This more difficult route would have been the Universe's attempt to teach her what she was able to learn relatively painlessly through therapy.

Realize that you are one with the Universe, that all that the Universe contains is within you, and begin now to take responsibility for what is happening. What you're likely to find is that you will begin to make the right choices. You'll find that you react to situations differently. Perhaps you normally get angry at your boss. This will change. It is difficult to be angry at someone whom you now realize represents a dark side of yourself that needs to be brought into the light.

As a result of this new attitude and outlook, you'll set in motion more healing for others and for yourself. You will permit your soul to develop by degrees in the areas where development is needed most. You know what needs work. What irritates you will be what you should concentrate upon. We tend to dislike in others what we subconsciously dislike on ourselves.

Forgive yourself and others

It is a divine law that if one does not forgive, then one is led to the other, for in reality that other person is us. What we have failed to do is to forgive our selves.

Release the anger. Forgive others. Forgive yourself. Forgive your parents. Forgive your siblings. If we begin to see the situations in our life as opportunities to practice forgiveness, like the angels we will be lighter.

In the words of George Roemisch, "Forgiveness is the fragrance of the violet which still clings fast to the heel that crushed it. Forgiveness is the broken dream which hides itself within the corner of the the mind, oft called forgetfulness so that it will not bring pain to the dreamer."

The Affirmation for Acceptance below, when said in multiples of 3, 9, 27, 36 times with heartfelt desire to undo errors in judgment, will assist you in healing your soul. May you have the courage to accept yourself and forgive others so that your soul can heal and soar like an eagle.

AFFIRMATION FOR ACCEPTANCE*

I AM FORGIVENESS ACTING HERE,
CASTING OUT ALL DOUBT AND FEAR,
SETTING MEN FOREVER FREE
WITH WINGS OF COSMIC VICTORY.
I AM CALLING IN FULL POWER
FOR FORGIVENESS EVERY HOUR;
TO ALL LIFE IN EVERY PLACE
I FLOOD FORTH FORGIVING GRACE.

*Source: "Heart, Head, and Hand Decrees," (released by Elizabeth Clare Prophet) Summit University Press, © 1987, page 4.

"For I am the Lord your God, the Lord of Hosts, who dried a path for you right through the sea, between the roaring waves. And I have put my words in your mouth and hidden you safe within my hand. I planted the stars in place and molded all the earth. I am the one who says, 'You are mine.'"

Isaiah 51:14-16 (The Living Bible)

CHAPTER FIVE
YOU ARE HERE FOR A PURPOSE

The author of a self-help book I recently read compares the earth to an elaborate theme park, such as Disney World. He believes we came to have experiences that aren't possible in the spiritual dimension. He also thinks that all minds are connected, and that the higher self of an individual, whom the author calls the "director" of the personal movie that we call our life, works behind the scenes with the higher selves of others to coordinate the comings and goings of different people and events. This is so we each can have the experiences we selected before we arrived.

It's an interesting idea, and there is no doubt some truth to it, but for me it falls short of a fully satisfying explanation of why we're here.

Others believe the earth is a school where we come to learn lessons that will lead to our personal evolution toward enlightenment.

There's truth in this, but I believe that it, too, falls a little short.

Many who call themselves Christians believe that we are here on earth to seek salvation. The earth provides a testing ground. If we pass, we will have everlasting life. If we fail, eternal damnation is our fate.

It's my personal policy to respect the beliefs of others, but I have to say, "Why would the Creator do this? He can create whatever he wants. Why wouldn't he make us perfect to begin with?"

To get at the true reality we are all part of, let's return to the analogy of Creation as a single living organism. Almost any medical doctor will say that the different parts of an organism exist to serve the whole. If it is true, as discussed in the last chapter, that all Creation is One, if it is true that each individual is a single facet, then each of us must exist to serve a purpose beyond our own enlightenment. Life must be more than a "movie" or "theme park" constructed for our personal amusement. We, like a kidney or a hand, must exist to serve the whole body. The whole body must be evolving, and us along with it. The entire universe and all humankind must be moving toward something bigger, greater and different than what now exists. This is where I come out. Of course, what I've written isn't an original idea. Many mystics and thinkers have said that, before a soul incarnates, it enters into a contract with the Universe to accomplish a particular mission or missions.

Think about it. Spend some time in meditation on the subject. Each person is different. Like snowflakes every one of us is unique. We are each a child of the Universe. We are each a cutting from the larger tree. Allowing our hang-ups or feelings of inferiority to hold us back, whether we developed them in a previous life or this one, is against the natural order. It is not what Creation intended.

The power of purpose

Deepak Chopra in *The Seven Spiritual Laws of Success* writes that underlying all creation exists a field of pure potentiality. This is divinity in its essential form. This potentiality takes on human form and, reflecting the same line of thinking I've just shared with you, becomes you and me and the woman next door — to fulfill different purposes. He says the word "dharma" is a Sanskrit word that means "purpose in life." Each person on this earth has a dharma that involves expressing the unique talent or combination of talents she was born with. She needs only to seek, and she will find the way it is intended she does this.

Dr. Chopra explains how important it is to instill thoughts such as these in children. He told his children from an early age that there was a reason why they were here, and that they would find what it was simply by being aware and getting in tune with their inner voice. He taught them how to meditate, and to "listen" in this way to a higher power. He told them he didn't want them to worry about getting the best grades in school or about going to the best colleges. All he wanted was for each child to seek how they best could serve humanity using the unique talents they possessed. Nevertheless, each of his children did get the best grades, did go to the best schools. Each is now financially self-sufficient, because they focused not on themselves but, rather, on what they are here to give.

All well and good, you say. But what happens if we didn't have Dr. Chopra as our parent? How do we discover this self that is in contact with the essence of divinity? How do we separate the personality part, the ego and its selfish desires and its fears, from the authentic higher self that dwells deep within? Most of us have a good deal of homework that has become backed up on us. We need to tackle it in order to catch up to the place we'd be if we'd had parents and teachers who were in tune with what now seems the true and logical reality of life.

Recognize your inner voices

We each have inner voices. The biggest problem is that we usually have several. Maybe many. And not all inner voices are the voice of the higher self. In fact, most are not. If an inner voice shouts at you, if it shames you, if it cajoles, nags or tries to persuade, it is NOT the voice of your higher self. In Chapter Six we will deal with this in more depth. But for now, simply consider that these are old tapes that your mind is playing. They might be reruns of your parents, teachers or siblings. They may be your own self-doubts. Turn your back on them. Flip the switch to "off." These tapes have outlived their usefulness.

The higher self, by contrast, is always calm and serene. Even in the middle of a hair-raising crisis, it will project serenity and confidence.

Don't be mistaken. The higher self can speak in a loud voice. It has never happened to me, but I've had friends say it has spoken to them with such volume, they actually turned around and looked to see if someone behind them had said something.

But it doesn't shout. It doesn't attempt to manipulate. Rather, it is matter-of-fact and wise. It has a calming effect. Even in the face of death.

The voice of the higher self

This calm and serene voice is not the only way the higher self communicates. It comes through to communicate with us in thoughts, insights, books, the Scriptures, nature, visions, dreams, circumstances — you name it. It comes in a thousand ways. When you see it or hear it or it gives you an insight, you'll know it's straight from the higher self because it "feels" authentic and true. It has an uplifting quality about it. It never ever has a "downer" quality.

In my own case I found the ability to communicate with my higher self through kinesiology/results therapy. I believe it is my purpose at this point in my life to share this technique with you.

In this new approach to healing the therapist does not go actively probing for a past life. Rather, the therapist uses muscle-testing in order to "carry on a conversation" with the individual's higher self. As previously explained muscle testing is a form of biofeedback that allows the therapist to bypass the ego and all its self-preservation techniques. In addition to kinesiology other new methodologies have emerged using the client-as-co-therapist approach.

Kinesiology/results therapy

In conventional therapy the therapist is the expert. The therapist tries to analyze every word for nuances and hidden meanings. Every facial gesture, every body movement and position, every inflection of the voice is considered and evaluated Every emotional reaction is scrutinized. Behavior patterns are painstakingly pieced together by the therapist, who then forms a diagnosis of what is troubling the individual.

In kinesiology/results therapy the client talks about an event or uses a physical technique to release emotional stress. When the client has had enough emotional release, as established by muscle-testing, the client is ready to help the therapist identify beliefs that need to be replaced.

The therapist reviews her session notes and decides which of the client's beliefs need to be addressed. The therapist then attempts to identify what new belief system should be used to replace the old.

The client's muscle again are tested to verify the system that has been identified is indeed what is needed. After the replacement, the new belief system is tested for verification that it has taken hold.

Unlike conventional therapists, the kinesiology/results therapist acts as a supportive teacher for what in effect is a client's self-therapy. When I have been a patient of a kinesiology/results therapist, I almost always walk away from a session feeling uplifted and strengthened. No one is unloading what may, in reality, be their own issues, judgments or hang-ups on me. My uniqueness has been honored. My higher self has communicated what I need at that time, and I feel good about it.

A therapist's notes record only a small fragment of what a client is actually experiencing. As a client myself, I've never shared with my therapist what in a romance novel might be called the really "juicy" parts. I save them for myself alone. I tell the therapist enough to let her know that I'm still grounded in the here and now. In truth the best insights are those that the client puts together herself. Because of this, it is important for the client to be alert to patterns. Patterns are like themes, such as the story behind Romeo and Juliet and West Side Story. Girl and boy from rival families or clans fall in love. It's impossible for them to be together, given their circumstances — making them star-crossed lovers. You can imagine all the problems that can come about as a result. The players may change but the story remains the same.

Whether they really are past lives, daydreams generated by your subconscious or memories plucked from the Universal Unconscious, your higher self has decided what it wants you to "remember" based on what you need to address in order to unload hang ups and fears. Your higher self wants you to move forward and to get going on what you came to earth to do. As a result, these past-life memories are likely to have themes. These themes are clues to what you need to work on. They probably point to the root of what's holding you back.

The therapist's notes — about what clients recall when they have a "memory" — don't have to go into a great deal of detail. Rather, they form a window through which the therapist can help identify beliefs that lead to unhappy situations. For example, if a person believes that all men are incompetent, that belief will be like a magnet. It will cause that individual to attract only incompetent men. Thus, a belief becomes reinforced by experience.

Beliefs are very powerful thoughts. As was written earlier, "thoughts are things." It is as though they have a life of their own, and will do anything to prove themselves to be true, even if what comes about is harmful to the one who holds the thoughts.

As one who has employed many different psychotherapies, I particularly like the techniques I'm sharing in this book, because they can be used without the aid of a trained therapist. They're safe, and can be used at your own speed. You ought to be able to gain at least general insights into your psyche, release much of what may be holding you back and integrate the shadow and suppressed aspects of yourself that surface. For particularly stressful events or traumas you should, of course, call upon a therapist for help and support.

You remember Mary. She had experiences that took place outside of sessions with me from which she learned a great deal. When it got "heavy," as Mary would describe it, she would come to me for assistance, and we'd both learn together.

Mary is a trained social worker, but her story could be anyone's. Her professional training did not factor into the way she went about learning her life lessons. I hope that her example will motivate readers to move quickly and easily through emotional pain in order to learn their own lessons. Her story, in a sense, is a gift. It teaches us that if we fail to explore a past remembrance that carried deep emotion with it, we may miss an important opportunity. Because of our denial, we may actually set ourselves up for another, far more difficult learning experience.

Accept your birthright

I should add, however, that "memories," such as the one that Mary experienced, normally do not surface until the higher self decides an individual is ready to deal with issues that will be raised. This is why it is so important to understand that you are here to accomplish something, and that you are a piece of the divine spark. You are worthy. You deserve peace of mind. You need it, and the Universe wants you to have it. You and the Universe are one.

Now you know that as a child of the Universe, as a drop of water in the larger ocean, all that exists in the Universe exists in you. What you must also come to accept is that this means both the good and the bad. Some of us may not be ready to face what we may consider to be the bad within us. We may not be able to accept that Hitler, for example, or Ted Bundy were also chips off the same block, and are part of our hologram. But if all is One, and I believe it is, then it follows that they are. This may not be a pleasant thought. But they are within you and me, no doubt well hidden in some shadowy corner. As long as we keep them in the shadow, they're going to jump out and bite us now and then. It's better to bring them into the open, accept that they are part of us and move on.

Accept all of you

What am I driving at? Simply this. You may have done some things in your life or in a past life that you're not so proud of. You must not berate yourself for the bad, any more than you should feel false pride about the good. You are a hologram of Creation, and everything that is imaginable and then some, good or bad, is part of Creation and, therefore, part of you. Accept this. Welcome it. Incorporate it into your being. Sense the power this knowledge brings. As a being of Creation who has been given freewill, you can choose which aspects of yourself to put in the driver's seat and which to keep in back. You have within you the potential to be another Mother Teresa or a Jeffrey Dahlmer. Which you choose is up to you.

Memories that will help you see where you need to direct your efforts will come when you are ready. Mary, for example, began by talking to me about her reactions to a movie. Her story should help all of us understand that what is not viewed with love and incorporated through forgiveness comes back to us — if not in one lifetime, then in the lifetime during which we are most ready for it. Her story shows how we treat others and relate to them is an indication of what is going on inside of us. We project and create on the outside what needs acceptance and healing within.

Some say that time is a dimension, and believe that there are an almost infinite number of dimensions. If what they believe is true, all our lives, past and future, may in reality be happening at once. If so, past life is actually concurrent life. Our focus is the present, but we are energy (matter = energy and energy = matter), and we are spirit. Energy is eternal. As every nuclear physicist knows, it cannot be created or destroyed. Therefore, we have always existed and always will.

How can this be? Why are we not aware of the eternal aspect of ourselves?

Gary Zukav, in his book *The Seat of the Soul,* explains that most of us operate almost exclusively through our ego selves and that the ego is limited in its perception to stimuli that arrive through one or more of the five senses. As an individual evolves and strives to get in touch with her soul or higher self through meditation and other means, she becomes "multi-sensory." Intuition becomes more developed. An awareness of the oneness of Creation dawns on the individual. Eventually, the person senses that all is one. She may not have arrived at an intellectual understanding of all Creation as one living organism, but she "knows" this through some mysterious sixth sense. Eternity actually may be glimpsed in what might be labeled an epiphany or religious experience.

When this happens, an individual has gotten in touch, however briefly, with her own soul and with all Creation. For a brief moment the two may actually have merged. My experience has been that following this experience, an individual often is totally transformed. In the past courage may have been lacking, but now that person is able to take hold of her life and find new courage in the knowledge that life is cyclical, that her life will continue forever and ultimately that all the hardship and evil will pass away. Good and truth will win out. You see, the soul and the soul alone knows the past and the future.

Care for your soul

But the soul, often referred to in the feminine as "she," is vulnerable. She is wounded by physical and emotional abuse, discordant music and violence, even violence as depicted in movies and of course, actual violence in relationships. In many ways the soul is like a child who lives inside us and seeks peace.

According to Zukav, the five-sensory personality must become aware of his or her intentions. Intentions are energy put into motion. Without awareness of these currents of energy, the personality will never be ready or able to experience reverence. Reverence is not an emotion. It is a way of being. It is perhaps the highest state of being that can be found in bodily form on earth. It is what you and I would do well to be striving for. The path to reverence is through a person's heart, which in reality is her feelings. These can be very subtle for many. The way may be opened through meditation. However it is reached, only an awareness of your feelings can truly open your heart.

A person who has found reverence through the opening of their heart becomes more than just a cuddly teddy bear. Having heart means bringing light to others where there is none. Having heart means looking compassionately upon evildoers, even while helping them change their minds so that they will change their deeds. When a person acknowledges her soul and comes to serve the soul, and by doing so a higher power, the experience allows that personality to become aligned. And the soul heals. The soul becomes an integrated whole.

The body is the instrument of the soul. And the condition of the body is often reflective of the condition of the soul. If the body is diseased, the soul must be in need of healing.

We can only get to the root cause of an illness through the soul itself. As Zukav asks, "If the piano player is sick, does it help to repair his or her piano?"

We must care for our souls in a loving manner, as we would care for our children. When the soul is empowered by God and knows it, the soul is fearless. It goes after the raging of the ego, the not-self (the things I do that I wish I would not do), and all other negative emotions and traits that would destroy life or the mission of others.

Knowing how a soul becomes splintered and diseased can help us know how to prevent its loss. Sometimes the soul is lost through the misuse of power. We give the soul away, for example, if we love someone so much that we permit them to misuse us, to physically or emotionally abuse us.

Sexual assault is more than a sexual act. It is an act of power and anger that invades the inner space and fragments the soul. Anything that increases the separation within a person from the God-source shatters the soul or diminishes its strength. Brutality shatters the soul, as does pain and irrationality, lying and blame. These are all poisons to the body.

If we verbally or physically abuse one another, our anger diminishes the soul, resulting in low self-esteem. We have permitted the soul to be trampled — to be frightened away.

Sister Francis in *Testimony of Light* says it this way:

> *I am aware too that in the last life experience I but repeated old struggles. None of it was new. No adventure into matter, into the exterior, is ever entirely fresh or untried. It has all been worked to its end perhaps hundreds of times before, though under different circumstances, perhaps in different worlds. I can not be sure of that yet, and it will be worked again until we, as souls, learn to 'carry the Light' with us, through our personalities. Freewill, the development of the logical mind, the illusions of the senses, all these tend to extinguish, or at least, to dim, the Light of Divinity. Now I perceive more clearly, for I am no longer cluttered by illusions, that the great purpose of his in matter is to illumine matter with Spirit.*
>
> *Time, as we reckoned it, does not exist here. Consciousness has taken its place. By the degree of consciousness of the Spirit can we measure the extent of the habitation of varying states in our onward progress.*
>
> *After the death of the physical body we gravitate to our right place; a mansion, a cottage, even a hovel, as we have earned. It is essential therefore to regard the experience, whilst in incarnation on the earth plane, as a preparation for this existence. Live Life in Eternity Now.*

In order to follow this advice, we must be a teacher to the soul. We must retrieve it. We must then find our purpose and begin to live it. Use the techniques outlined here to uncover the belief system that has hindered you. Resolve, also, to come to resolution with family members. Regardless of what family members did to you in the past, agree to disagree so that you can maintain your peace. When we do not maintain peace, we cannot magnetize peace back to ourselves. We cannot control other people; we can only control ourselves and thereby win our own soul back. It is the strength of love in our hearts that brings the fragments of the broken vase of our soul back together. It takes even greater love expanding from that heart of service to others to hold the pieces of the broken vase together, and mend the cracks till it is well again.

In short, collect the pieces of the soul wherever they may be. When you see your vase whole as if it had never been broken, you will be ready to embark on the next level of the journey, which is to find and live your purpose, to feel the joy of waking up on a Monday morning and bounding out of bed — bounding out of bed because you can't wait to get started doing what you absolutely love to do. You'll know that joy because you will take absolute responsibility for every decision you make, and the consequences of every decision. You'll know that joy because you'll be carrying out the mission you agreed upon before you came.

Seize the opportunity of life

Let me share a bit of ancient Oriental wisdom. "Life is an opportunity, not an obligation." Believe me, when you have your soul back in one piece, you'll start seeing it that way.

In another place and another time, a very wise young man gave people some advice about following their hearts and fulfilling their soul purpose, as opposed to chasing the money they thought they needed in order to feed and clothe themselves. He told them to look around at nature, at the birds of the air, for example. Birds don't worry. They don't store up grain for the winter, they don't plant, reap or sow. They just do what birds do, what nature meant them to do, and they get along just fine.

This wise young man probably was standing in a field at the time. He asked his followers to look around, and he said, "See how the lilies of the field grow. They do not labor and spin. Yet I tell you that not even Solomon in all his glory was dressed as one of these."

What was he talking about?

The young man was trying to communicate that the lilies of the field are doing what they were meant to do. They are doing what nature intended for them. They aren't working at it. They don't "labor or spin." They aren't even trying, yet they are doing it very well.

The people he was talking to were worried about having enough to eat and whether they would have clothes to wear, just as you may at times be worried about having enough to eat and clothes to wear. The wise young man pointed out that these simple lilies of the field, by doing what they were meant to do, were dressed in such glorious outfits that they would put even Solomon to shame.

Who was Solomon?

Solomon had been a king of Israel, a king of the Jews, a long time before this wise young man spoke. Solomon's was a glorious period. During his reign the people of Israel had their most prosperous days. Never before, never since had their land been so large, so rich and so peaceful as it was then. The people our wise young man was speaking to instantly would have known who Solomon was, because he had been the wisest, wealthiest and most honored king in their entire history — yet even Solomon in all his glory was not dressed as magnificently as simple lilies of the field, doing what nature intended for them.

You are part of nature, just like the lilies of the field. Like the lilies of the field, it was not an accident that you were born. Like the lilies of the field, you have something you were intended to do. You have a calling. You may not now know what that calling is, not at this moment, but you do have it. You were born with a special gift, talent or combination of talents that no one else possesses in precisely the same way. Your true and intended destiny is to put those talents or that gift to work in a way, or ways, that will benefit others.

This is what nature had in mind. This is what your soul had in mind before you were born. Whether or not you now realize it, this is your deep and unwavering desire. You need to get in touch with and listen to that desire. It exists deep in your heart.

Spend some time in meditation asking yourself what gift you have. What can you do better than anyone? What do you enjoy? How would you like to spend your time and your life? What do you have to give? Ask the Universe to tell you. Then be on the lookout for an answer. Keep your eyes open. Remember that the higher self or soul speaks and communicates in a thousand different ways. My experience has been that an answer will come.

Once you discover your calling, begin to pursue it, and you will know that you are at last "on purpose." By following that purpose you will help others, and in turn you will help yourself. This is the natural way. It is nature's way. You, like the lilies of the field, were meant to do your thing, to do what you do best, what no one else can do quite the way you do. This is why Jesus spoke those words about the lilies of the field 2,000 years ago, and why I offer them to you.

TWIN FLAME

As a fiery ovoid, we were one -- soul of soul and heart of heart.

As an eternal flame burning as one, we wanted to come to Earth.
Our Father divided us into two parts so that each would learn
the lessons of life.

Yet, along the way, we made choices.
Choices based on lust not love.
Choices that separated us from each other.
Choices that separated us from our God source.

Soul of my soul, where are you now?
All the other lovers are counterfeit.
I desire only you.
I choose only you.

It is only you who is me.
For you, my twin flame -- are heart of my heart, soul of my soul.

I sent my Soul through the invisible, some letter of the afterlife to spell, and by and by my Soul returned to me, and answered, I myself am Heaven and Hell.

— Omar Khayyam (c.1048-c.1122 A.D.)

CHAPTER SIX
LET YOUR LIFE BE INFORMED BY YOUR SOUL

At present if you are like most people, your soul takes a backseat in your life. Rather, your life and thoughts are informed by your ego. This is not a bad thing. Nor is it good. It is the way things now are, but not how they have to be. You can free yourself. You can give yourself wings, but to do so, how you and your ego interact may need modification and adjustment.

The role of the ego

Many thoughtful men and women have come to the conclusion that we must push the ego aside in order to get in touch with the soul, but in my opinion they have misunderstood the essential nature of the ego. Our ego creates and maintains our boundaries, our sense of where we end and others begin. Without it we indeed would perceive ourselves as All-That-Is, or God, just as a newborn in his crib may consider himself to be the center of the Universe. We must have a clear understanding of our self as a separate being before a sense of oneness is viable or healthy. Otherwise, we may think we are justified in doing exactly as we please, treating the world and others as extensions of ourselves, existing to serve us and to do our bidding. Narcissism is the term psychologists use to identify the mental condition brought about by the arrested development of the ego. Antisocial behavior often is the result.

A healthy, properly-developed ego, on the other hand, allows us to be open to spiritual development and vision. It allows us to open ourselves to our soul. The ego must grow as we grow, so that we become secure in our sense of self. Properly developed, the ego can become the container that can house the soul without threatening mental, emotional or physical collapse. Those who possess underdeveloped egos are threatened by contact with the higher self or soul because of buried fears. As previously mentioned, the ego's first job is self-preservation. A weak ego fears the higher self or soul will swallow or annihilate the ego if allowed full rein.

An underdeveloped ego is also "egotistical." It wants to take credit for whatever it can, when in reality it may be responsible for very little. Nevertheless, it will do all in its power to puff itself up, even to the extent of denying the possibility of anything beyond itself. It may, for example, do all in its power to cut you off from communication with a higher power. If threatened, the ego can turn on you and bring the action to a stop by pushing just the right buttons. To prevent this from happening, you may need to undergo some deprogramming.

Reprogram your ego

Next time you begin to get all jumbled up and in a dither, slow down and consider what triggered the reaction. Did your temper flare? Why? Why was it so important things go your way? If you retrace what you felt back to its cause, in most cases you will come to a particular variety of fear. It has been said that only two fears are of an instinctive nature: the fears of high places and loud noises. The others were acquired in this life or another. Remember this: Whatever you have acquired, you can dispose of.

Just about every fear that can be imagined can be categorized under one of six headings: 1) poverty (or failure), 2) criticism, 3) ill health, 4) loss of love, 5) old age and 6) death.

I've listed the fear of poverty (failure) first because in many ways it can be the most debilitating. To quote Edgar Cayce again, "Thoughts are things." As a result of this fear, which is in reality only a thought buried in your subconscious, traits develop in you that bring it about. For example, are you a procrastinator? An underlying fear of failure is probably the root cause and can be counted upon to produce that result.

Are you overly cautious? Do you see the negative side of every circumstance or stall for the "right time" before taking action? Do you worry (that things will not work out), have doubts (generally expressed by excuses or apologies about why you probably won't be able to perform), suffer from indecision (which leads to someone else or circumstances making the decision for you)?

Are you indifferent? This generally manifests as laziness or a lack of initiative, enthusiasm or self-control.

Step back and listen for internal voices that say "can't" or "don't" or "won't" or "too risky" or "why bother?" Move your point of awareness, or consciousness, outside your head. Place it on your shoulder or just above your head. Observe. Listen to the thoughts running through your head.

Are they destructive?

Shoo them away.

Whether you are the president of a nation or a company or a bum on skid row the only thing over which you have absolute control is your thoughts.

You may say, "I can't control what thoughts pop into my head." True. You may not be able to control what thoughts arise, but you can decide whether to discard a thought or keep it. You can decide that it is counterproductive and trash it, or you can turn it over and over in your mind, nurture it and let it grow. Remember that what you focus on expands. Whatever thoughts you keep will expand, too, and eventually manifest. The bad and the good.

Beginning now, each time you catch yourself with a negative thought, a thought that says, "You can't," "It's not possible," "Maybe someone else but not me," get rid of it.

But you say, "I'm poor, I'm not a good student, I'm not a good salesperson, I'm in the lower third of productivity... "

You are what you are because of your thoughts. Your higher self wants the best for you, but your ego is holding you back because of its programming.

If what I've been writing about here is a serious problem for you, go out and buy some self-help tapes that will plant positive thoughts in your mind in place of the negative ones. Play them to and from work and before you go to sleep at night. Use self-hypnosis tapes. Play them over and over for at least a month. Get all that junk out of your head and replace it with thoughts that are positive.

How about the other fears? They're to be discarded, too. If you suffer from fear of criticism, for example, it probably came about as a result of a parent or sibling who constantly tore you down in order to build himself up. The telltale signs of the fear of criticism are worry about what others will think, lack of poise, self-consciousness and extravagance.

Why extravagance? Because one of your inner voices keeps telling you that you need to keep up with the Jones. You must rid yourself of it. Who cares what people say?

Let's take a closer look at the fear of criticism. Maybe this one, as well as others, stems from a past life. There have been places and times in history when what others thought was worth worrying about. Suppose, for example, you are the incarnation of someone who was hanged in Salem, Massachusetts, back in 1692. Suppose you were able to run the farm without a man around. Can you imagine the talk that would have generated? Such a thing wasn't possible, or so your neighbors might have believed, without the use of witchcraft.

In that day and time the opinions of others mattered a great deal. They could well lead to an unpleasant and untimely death.

What about today?

Maybe if you live in a particular country outside of the industrialized world, you might have to watch out. If you do, it's doubtful you'd be reading this book. In some of them that alone could land you in jail.

In just about every developed nation what others think or don't think of you or anyone else is their problem. Yet worrying about what they think can cause a great deal of misery, create karma which will have to be worked out and cause interference between you and your soul. It can block communication.

So much for the fear of criticism. How about the fear of ill health?

Remember this: What you worry about, think about, and focus on is also what happens. That knowledge alone should be enough for you to do whatever necessary to unload this insidious fear.

Have you ever noticed that it's the people who talk about illness, worry about illness, are preoccupied with this or that possible illness, think they feel a pain here or there or were exposed to some germ, who are precisely the people who stay sick most of the time?

Suppose you're a tennis buff. Next time you're in a big match and it's close and you arrive at a crucial point and your opponent is serving holler out, "You're playing great today, Morris. Don't blow it. This is a big point coming up. Try not to double-fault."

Watch him double-fault. It's dirty. It will create negative karma. But it works.

How about the fear of the loss of love? This one manifests in the form of jealousy and also is self-fulfilling. The person you try so hard to hang onto feels smothered, and you end up pushing him away. Be yourself, instead. Give him room. If he leaves you, he would have done so anyway. What we all need, and what you will achieve by following the advice in this book, is a sense of worth that isn't dependent on a relationship with someone else.

Next? The fear of old age.

This one is closely connected to the fear of ill health and the fear of poverty, because these are the conditions a person actually is concerned about, deep down. The power of suggestion is at work here, too. If you *think* you're too old to do this or that, you will indeed be too old to do this or that.

Consider this. I have a friend, a man, who is fifty years old and has a one-year-old daughter. His daughter is comprised of the same flesh and blood as he and wife. The cells that comprise her body grew from his sperm and mother's egg. She's the continuation of an unbroken chain of division that dates back to the first life on earth. All life everywhere you look is approximately the same age. Billions of years. Why should your flesh and blood be old, and the one-year-old's be young? Why? Your body gets old and decrepit because you expect it to get old and decrepit. Sure, maybe an enzyme is involved in the aging process, but it's your thoughts that trigger the release of this enzyme.

Forget about your age. Banish any thoughts about it.

Okay. Now we've come to that final bugaboo, the fear of death.

If you've been paying attention up to this point in this book, you now realize you have nothing to fear. You are energy. Energy is neither created nor destroyed. Your soul is eternal. You are eternal.

Your soul is eternal

Consider the millions who have had near-death experiences and are no longer afraid to die. Having done it once already, they now know they'll be greeted by loved ones who have gone before. They look forward to being bathed once again in the all-encompassing light. Many have described this light as total, unconditional love. Can you imagine anything better than that?

Most who have experienced NDEs no longer expect to experience pain. It has been reported by many that the spirit exits the body the precise instant it looks as though death is inevitable.

Only a handful who have come back from the other side had hell-like experiences while they were there. It is true that they, indeed, are worried about what they may encounter after death. These folks need to know what already has been made clear to you. Each of us creates his or her own reality. We experience what we expect to experience. We experience what we think we deserve. In the physical world this takes time. In the nonphysical we create it instantly. If we expect hell, the hell we believe we deserve is the hell we will get. If we expect heaven, our vision of heaven is what we will have.

Anyone who has ever had a lucid dream will understand this. Such a dream is one in which a person realizes she's dreaming. As soon as a lucid dreamer is aware she is dreaming, she can begin to compose the dream. She can determine the players, the surroundings, the action. What happens if she wants to fly over the Grand Canyon? She simply "thinks" this. Fly over is what she will do, no airplane required.

Be a lucid dreamer

One goal of this chapter is to wake you to the reality that you are a dreamer in the big dream of life, and that you can make this dream you are having lucid. Until now you may have thought you were at the mercy of conditions outside yourself. You may have thought that you have either been lucky or unlucky, or that chance has brought you where you are. This isn't true. You've brought yourself to this spot, consciously or unconsciously. If this is not where you want to be, it's because your ego self was programmed incorrectly. It's because you're out of touch with your higher self or soul. Perhaps you hear snippets from it every now and then, but you ignore what it's trying to say because of other voices. These other voices beat it back with words such as "can't," "don't," "shouldn't," "too risky." Those are the words of your ego. Your higher self wants so much more for you and knows so much more is possible.

Begin the deprogramming process now. There's absolutely no reason to wait. Begin today to bring your ego self and your higher self, or soul, together. Allow them to work in harmony. Once you do, you'll be in position to enter Nirvana, what others call the Kingdom of God. You'll know on a gut level the connectedness of all things. You'll determine your surroundings and the outcome of each and every adventure. You'll be a lucid dreamer in the dream of life.

"Sounds great," you say. "Now, tell me how to do that again."

You have to quiet the ego. You've got to deal with its campaign of terror. And the simplest way is to observe what's going on inside your head with detachment, as though you were standing on the outside. Imagine your ego as a fearful child who needs reassurance, or as a student who needs to be educated and brought along. This involves becoming aware of what your conscious mind has abdicated to your unconscious, and this is where kinesiology/ results therapy can help. You see, if you aren't where you want to be, it's your unconscious that's chauffeured you there. The past life "memories"that surface in therapy can bring to light what's holding you back.

Slow down. Put on the brakes. Relax. Meditate about your condition. Think about destructive behaviors that you repeat. Let thoughts and memories bubble up. Consider them. View them with detachment. What are the recurring patterns? Why are the characters not able to achieve what what they consciously would like to. If you can figure that out, you probably can figure out how you got where you are.

Once you realize this, you can educate your ego. Explain what it's been doing and ask it to stop. Let it know the fears it propagates aren't helping matters. They're hurting. Strengthen your ego to the point where you will be able to bring it in touch with your higher self — where, in essence, it will be dissolved in love. Otherwise, your ego will make a concerted effort to stop the action by drowning out all communication.

The higher self or soul is that part that connects you with the Eternal. It is the individual dreamer who is in contact with the other dreamers and the Big Dreamer, the One Life of which each of us is part. It is that part of us which provides a sense of meaning and value. It is what comes through us to create a sense of intimacy with another human being or another creature. The soul or higher self is reaching out to us when we feel the need to know the meaning of life or our own individual life. It is reaching out when we feel a hunger to experience our connection to the All. It is reaching out when we contemplate our mortality. It is the part of you that led you to this book.

The soul or higher self is most apparent when we are in a

period of transition. This may be during one of the seven-year cycles of our maturation; it may be when a child is born; when the death of a friend or loved one occurs; or in the period preceding our own physical death. Many cultures and virtually all spiritual brotherhoods have rituals and myths to aid in and soften these transitions. The lack of rituals and myths, the relative lack of regard for the spiritual dimension in our secular society, can make these passages difficult and lonely.

The techniques that now will be discussed are not meant to take the place of these rituals and myths. The aid and comfort they give can be one of the major benefits of your participation in a circle of others on the path. The techniques that follow are meant to provide you with practical, day-to-day methods for growing closer to your higher self with the ultimate goal of uniting this part of you with your ego to form a true, undivided Self.

When this occurs, the pot at the end of the rainbow will have been reached. You will experience a sense of wholeness as though you have arrived home at the end of a long journey. Your soul will soar. Your life will be transformed by a new principle that is in accordance with the order and objectives of the Universe. You will be led to a life of abundance, not necessarily of money or possessions, but in the form of the fulfillment and joy of existing in the flow. You will be led to a life of freedom you did not think possible. You will be aided and guided by unseen hands. You will be in a position to choose, because you will sense the outcome of your actions before you take them. You will bring the course of your life into harmony with your destiny. You will have reached a state of enlightenment.

Enlightenment is the natural state

All this sounds very grand and godlike but the truth is, enlightenment is our natural state. It is the state of all creatures in the wild. They also are guided by the the natural forces of the One Life. The higher self or the soul of swallows brings them back to Capistrano on the same day every year; it directs the herds of wildebeest across the African plains. It guides the migration of whales.

Man was the same as the other animals of nature before the mythical Garden of Eden. He remained fully in touch with the One Life, guided by instincts and higher forces. To put it another way, he was at one with God. By becoming self-conscious, however, by becoming aware of himself as separate and apart, he pulled the plug that connected him. What he believed himself to be became his reality, just as what you believe yourself to be is your reality. Man and woman no longer believed they were connected to God, and this belief became true for them. They indeed were separate. They were now capable of error, laziness and self-centeredness, and could not help but make mistakes and go astray.

Nowadays, you and I and a growing number of our fellow humans are arriving at the end of a long journey. We are nearing the completion of the period in our evolution, both as a species and as individuals, when it was necessary to concentrate our efforts on the development of the ego portion of our psyches. Wild animals such as birds or deer have no actual egos. They are plugged into a state of oneness with others of their species and the field. Our egos, which create and maintain our sense of separateness, have prevented this for all but the most advanced of our species. Until now. Now our goal must be to maintain our separate identities while simultaneously reuniting with our higher selves, or souls. When this is done, the last stage of our evolution in the physical world will be accomplished. Our journey on the earth will be complete.

Recognize your intuition

Most of us have been conditioned since birth to discount what is often described as intuition. As a result we've developed a habit of not listening to the voice of our higher self. If we are to reconnect, the first step is to acknowledge that intuition is real, that our higher selves exist and that it is possible for us to be in touch.

Not everyone receives intuitive insights or messages from their higher self in the same way. Some hear voices. The reception of extrasensory signals in the form of words, a sound or some from of language is called Psychic Hearing. It can be subtle, similar to what one hears in his mind when one talks to himself. It also can be loud and clear the way my friend experienced it. But, as I have previously written, it is never a voice that cajoles or attempts to manipulate.

Another way messages are received is called Psychic Vision or clairvoyance. This is a form of ESP that expresses itself as a picture, symbol or visual impression. Traditionally, it is associated with receiving visual insights either through meditation or in dreams. You probably are aware of psychics who help police by visualizing the scene of the crime or the location of the body. You may have had experiences with clairvoyance and not realized it. Have you ever had, for example, a mental image of an old friend, and then received a phone call or letter from that person?

Psychic Intuition, an instantaneous *sense of knowing,* is the most common form of reception. Degrees of this exist, ranging from a fleeting snippet that occurs spontaneously, to a permanent gut-level realization, a sense of knowing that continuously flows. The ultimate state is one in which the receiver "knows" himself to be Creation, All-That-Is, The One Life. I've had glimpses of this. I doubt anyone remains in it long; although some practitioners of yoga may approach a continuous state. It may take years of working at it, but I believe for most an ongoing connection that gives moment-by-moment guidance is possible, and a realistic goal. Not that we should discard the rational mind. It has its place. We simply need to recognize its limitations.

Our rational mind can be compared to a computer. It can sort the data (anything you have read or experienced), cross tab, analyze and spit out an answer. Unfortunately, no matter how competent your mental computer is, the answer may not be correct because the analysis is limited to the data your mind had to work with. This is not to say it isn't of value. It is probably all we need to make the right decisions most of the time. It tells us red light means stop, green light means go, don't touch a hot stove, one and one make two. A quick scan of one's database is enough. But your higher self should be consulted on the big issues because it isn't limited in any way. It is plugged into the infinite knowledge of the Universe. It has direct access to the Collective Unconscious.

Trust your higher self

Let's talk about how to cultivate a relationship. Like any relationship, it needs to begin with trust. As we've seen, the ego is terrified of losing control. Yet your ego must feel confident enough to allow your higher self to come though. The way I've done this is by convincing myself (my ego) that I don't have control, anyway. As much as I'd like, I cannot have control no matter how hard I try. Nothing is in my control except my thoughts. To believe otherwise is self-delusion. I have come to believe that the old saying is true, "Anything a person feels he must control, in reality controls him."

Start now and slowly ease into this new way of life. You might begin by setting aside a few minutes every day simply to daydream. Call this your quiet time. Dedicate up to a half-hour at least once, and twice a day if you can, from now on. It can be the most productive and important time in each twenty-four hours.

Sit back and relax or lie down. Allow yourself to enter a state of consciousness that's different from what you're used to during normal waking hours. You might get a tape or two on meditation to help you relax, but for the first week or so don't meditate. Daydream. This may be enough by itself to create the condition for insights to come through. Think of a quiet place, perhaps somewhere out in nature, where the temperature is perfect. Perhaps there's a blue sky and a gentle breeze. Allow yourself to go into a kind of trance, to drop to a deeper level of consciousness. Let your mind go wherever it takes you.

You may find that you begin identifying your true purpose and mission in life. Daydreams often are fantasies about who we really are or what we can be. They may be closer to the truth than what you thought was the truth until now. They may actually be memories from past lives. They may be your higher self's way of telling you what you need to be aware of and work on. They may reveal the destructive patterns that need to be erased.

When you reach a point where you are comfortable doing this, ask yourself what you would do if you could expand to your full potential. What is your bliss? What do you truly love?

I'm not talking about your ego's desire to sit on the beach and read a romance novel. I'm talking about how you would like to be involved in life, not watch it mosey by.

Spend quiet time each day

I've found that some people have a regular quiet time and do not realize it. It might be when they exercise or jog. It could be when they get up early in the morning and have a quiet cup of something hot to drink.

No matter when or how you elect to spend time getting in touch, ask yourself, how do your fantasies connect with the circumstances into which you were born? What games did you play as a child? How did you entertain yourself? Have you any interests that go back as far as you can remember?

Are you now doing what you like? Does what you do help others in some way? With your background and training what could you do? If you could have whatever you want, be whatever you want, what is it? How would this help others?

Do this each day for several days. What themes recur? Write them down. A pattern will emerge. Keep at it. What's it telling you about what needs to be discarded? What's it telling you about your destiny or calling?

Get rid of the former and develop the latter into a vision. Whatever this entails at first may seem impossible, but this could simply be your ego talking. Don't let it get in the way just because it's terrified. Stroke it. Tell it you're not going to quit your day job. Not this week, anyway. It is quite possible you may decide to modify your vision as you proceed. But by all means, do not begin by watering it down because of the seemingly "practical" voice of your ego. Your higher self already has the end result in mind. Let it help you bring this into focus.

The higher self knows how your vision can be achieved. Allow yourself to be shown the way. Ask for guidance in your daily quiet time. Sometimes the required information will come immediately. Often it will not. Be patient, an answer is on the way. It may arrive in several days or even a week later.

In general woman are able to get in touch with their higher self or intuition more readily than men. This is the source of the "wives' tale" of women's intuition. The reason is, in our culture women usually are in closer touch with their emotions. Intuition is a kind of emotion or "feeling." The truth is that intuition is of the right brain, and men as well as women can access it.

Feeling what emotions are communicating is one way to "listen" to your soul.

Ask for answers

Often I'll ask a question of my higher self at night before I go to sleep. If possible, I phrase the question so that a "yes" or "no" answer will give me the information that I need. I conclude by saying, "When I wake up tomorrow, let me realize the best course. Give me a sense of knowing." This almost always works for me. I never make an important decision without doing this first.

You may be wondering, "How can I tell if my higher self is telling me something or if it's some other part of me?" Many different feelings and conflicts are going on within me at any given time.

We've already discussed how to identify the flak thrown up by your ego. This revolves around worry and is usually fear-based. Disregard it. It has nothing to do with your higher self. Your higher self is never worried, does not know the meaning of fear. Nor is it the part of you that judges or says you must follow the rules. Communication from the higher self has a lightness to it, a sense of "This is right." It is not an addictive voice, either, one that says you need alcohol or drugs or some other person or a new car or a mink coat or membership in the country club to make you happy.

Recognize the still, small voice

If it has a sense of urgency to it, it probably has to do with some earth-bound fear or addiction. When you are bombarded with this kind of interference, release it. Let it float away. Go under this flak. Messages from your higher self have to do with what is right in the long run. This is always the case. For example, if you ask for the answer to a short-term problem, you'll get an answer that will serve the long haul. The result is, you may not understand at the time why you are led in a given way, but when you look back, you will. You'll see it had to do with inner things, with what is of true value, not with what will remain forever on the physical plane.

Being guided daily by my higher self has become a way of life for me, but is not something I expect you'll be willing to plunge into. Nor do you need to. Ease into it a day at a time. Try making minor decisions to test how it feels. For example, suppose you go to a party, and a feeling says this is not where you want to be. Your ego may counter with, "You can't leave. What would people think?"

Leave. Go home or wherever your inner voice directs you. When you get there, calm yourself. Check your feelings. If you were following higher guidance, you'll feel light, more alive. You'll have energy. Learn to recognize this feeling. In the future, even after you've made a big, potentially life-changing decision, you'll experience this same sense of buoyancy if you're following your higher self. If you are not, you'll feel drained, blocked, maybe even depressed, and it's time to reconsider.

As you work at listening to and practice following these messages, you'll find they get stronger. After awhile, it will become easier to sort out the ego-based voice, and to recognize communication from a higher source. Start with matters that aren't all that important and allow your confidence to build. If you persevere, you'll come to a point when you will be willing to allow your life to be guided in this way.

I won't try to tell you this whole business isn't scary at first. But once you start down this path, you won't want to turn back. You'll experience a new sense of freedom. I like to think of it as a great adventure. It really is better than Disney World.

Perhaps right now, today, you feel a sense of frustration with your life. You know something's wrong, that you'd be happier doing something else, but you don't know what. Begin consulting with your higher self. Ask to be shown the way. You can be confident things will change. There can be no other result. Your ego self may be terrified of this. Change can be very threatening. But tell your ego to hang on and trust. Your higher self is a gung-ho type that knows no fear, but in the long run, it isn't going to lead you astray.

Ask for awareness, a sense of knowing what you should do next. You might ask at night, as I often do, or during your daily quiet time. You may receive an image, a feeling or an answer in words right on the spot. You may draw a blank. If so, go about your business but expect an answer. Trust that it's on its way. It may come in a dream. It might come from outside yourself. You are part of the One Life, remember? Your extended body and mind is the Universe itself. The answer can come from anywhere. Be attentive.

Look: the answers can be anywhere

For me answers that come from outside my local body and mind usually arrive in written form. A phrase or paragraph in a book I'm reading will seem to stand out. The medium could be almost anything: a fortune cookie, a comic strip, the Bible, Dear Abby. Whatever it is will strike a cord, and have meaning for me and my situation that the author probably did not have in mind.

How does this work for me on a day-to-day basis? If a question or problem occurs in the morning while I'm working, when lunch comes I'll check my feelings to see if a trip to the library or a bookstore seems indicated. If so, I'll walk in and go to whatever section or shelf feels right, take a book from the shelf and open it at random. More often than not, the answer will be on that page. If not, I'll flip a few pages and look again. If the answer isn't there, I'll try another book. Seldom do I pick up more than three.

A friend tells me his answers usually come from other people. It could be something the preacher says in a sermon on Sunday. Or my friend might be engaged in a conversation at work about something totally unrelated, and a sentence or phrase a person says will jump out at him. He has his answer. The meaning for him may have nothing to do with what was being said.

Ask your higher self to direct you to a better life. Let it show you step by step. Don't try to force it. Don't make yourself make decisions. Just let things take place. If you allow yourself to be guided, things will happen. Remain flexible. Trust. Things probably will not occur the way you expect, nor will you end up where you thought at the outset your higher self was taking you. If you go down a path only to find a dead end, look around for the open door. You'll find it. You were led down that path because that's where the door is.

Your higher self knows what it's doing. It won't let you starve. At times things may look bleak, though, so be prepared. For example, you may wonder what's taking so long. Your higher self may seem to take delight in cutting things close. Its scheduling often seems just in the nick of time, but in reality its timing is perfect.

No mistakes, only lessons

The question is bound to arise: Can your higher self make a mistake? Can it lead you down the metaphorical primrose path? The answer is an emphatic, "No." It cannot make a mistake. You may make a mistake interpreting it, but your higher self knows what it's doing. It's plugged into the One Life.

But don't take my word for it. Be cautious until you are one hundred percent confident in your ability to understand what you are being told. Ask for confirmation. Ask for reassurance. Ask and you will receive. But do not ignore your intuition. If you do not pay attention to it, if you do not move at least cautiously in the direction it is pushing you, you'll become blocked. Listening to your higher guidance and learning to understand is like any skill. The more you do it, the better you get at it and the easier it becomes. Like anything, use it or lose it. If you happen to make a wrong turn, the mistake will not be a disaster if you honestly were trying do the right thing. Your higher self and the forces of Grace will come to your aid in such situations.

Write down your fears. Turn these statements around into positive affirmations. "My needs are being taken care of." "My life is getting better and better." Repeat them to yourself whenever the negative thought reoccurs. And keep in mind what Jesus said:

> *And do not set your heart on what you will eat or drink; do not worry about it. For the pagan world runs after such things, and your Father knows that you need them. But seek his kingdom, and these things will be given to you as well.*
>
> — Luke 12:29-31

It helps to have at least one other person you can talk to about your fears. This should be someone who is also following the path laid down by his higher self. This is where a good therapist who is in tune with the teachings of this book can make a big difference.

The person you select should not be a family member, however, or a co-worker or anyone who still has his own ego fears to clear. He only will reflect back to you the fears you are trying to unload.

Affirmations for Transfiguration

I do my best.
My best is good enough.
I am perfect in my imperfection.
I take responsibility for my own well-being.
I take responsibility for their own-well being.
Others take responsibility for their own well-being.
Others take responsibility for their own happiness.
I allow others to take responsibility for their own happiness.
I respect who I am.
I respect others for who they are.
Other respect me for who I am.
I respect my wants and needs.
I have everything I need within me.
I trust the future.
I trust the unknown.
I trust my own knowing.
I trust others.
Others trust in me.
I make choices that lead me to my highest good.
My actions lead me to my highest good.
I am my own approval.
I accept and appreciate who I am.
I accept and appreciate who others are.
Others accept and appreciate who I am.

"For He will give His angels charge of you,
to guard you in all your ways."

— Psalms 91:11

CHAPTER SEVEN
USE YOUR BODY TO REJOIN MIND AND SOUL

There are no accidents in this universe. A reason is behind every event. What will help our soul to heal and become whole is to understand the reason and learn the lesson that often underlies an event, emotion or memory. Then we are in position to incorporate this new knowledge and move on.

The last chapter encouraged you to begin allowing your life to be informed by your soul. This will deal more specifically with techniques you can employ to facilitate a connection between you, your spiritual essence and the Universal Mind.

We are each part of One Life. Nowhere are we more likely to comprehend and connect with this reality than when surrounded and engulfed by nature. Outdoors, away from the concrete of the city, we find ourselves quite literally located in the very center of the Universal Mind. Often we need only to open our eyes and our hearts to feel this. The realization cascades throughout our entire being.

Meditate in nature

Spend time in nature every day if possible, meditating, observing. Allow yourself to be filled with a sense of awe at the beauty of a sunset or a mountain vista. Realize that what you behold is your extended body. What is at the root of all you see is the very intelligence that resides within you. The "urge to become" that is behind the unfolding of the trees and plants in spring is also inside you. You and Nature are One.

You may wish while in this environment to seek out "memories" that will bring about a greater understanding of who you are. One man recounted to me that upon observing fish swimming beneath the surface of a creek, a memory suddenly flooded his awareness of passing through many forms, from single-cell creature, to fish, to reptile, to small furry animal, to his present state of Homo sapiens.

Why shouldn't a memory of this be possible? As an embryo in his mother's womb, his body did pass through each of these states as it developed. The cells in his body and his DNA can be traced backward in time along an unbroken chain to that simple one-cell animal. Similarly, his awareness evolved through various levels and degrees of comprehension to reach what it is today. In a very real way this man experienced the ultimate in time travel. While many in my presence have recalled past lives, this man recalled the entire journey, in summary form, from his emergence as life in the primordial sea to his present incarnation as a family man and office worker of the modern age.

Time travel "memories" are important, not because someone was once a queen or a president or Napoleon, but because time travel can teach us lessons that can allow us to heal. The process can take years. Sometimes the reason is not readily apparent; when this is the case, the full lesson has yet to be learned. If time travelers fail to pay attention and do their "homework" by finding meaning that brings personal growth, the memories will return in one form or another.

To become whole you will have to deal with issues that were put into motion at points along the way of your journey from the primordial sea to the current day. In addition to kinesiology/

results therapy, several methods exist to facilitate this process. One is whole brain learning, or brain integration.

Some researchers tell us that the left side of the brain is more logical, sequential and linear, while the right brain takes a more holistic approach to experiencing and processing reality. The left brain likes the detail. The right sees the entire picture. By using the whole brain we can comprehend so much more than if we rely exclusively on only one of its hemispheres.

Whole brain exercises

One approach to facilitate comes from Dennison's *Educational/ Kinesiology* and is known as "Brain Gym." It involves a cross-motor activity mentioned at the beginning of this book called the cross-crawl.

Glenn Doman, a physical therapist, found that his work had little effect on children who had suffered brain damage. Those who had physical therapy while in the hospital and those who did not performed about the same in the long run. In his quest to discover why, he researched how babies learn and develop. Doman found, for example, that newborn babies would move across their cribs or the floor in a cross-crawl fashion. By studying the children of different cultures, Doman soon found that this movement, the cross-crawl, was critical for brain development. It involves a hand or arm being moved simultaneously with an opposing leg.

Dr. Dennison, a former associate of Doman, established the Educational Kinesiology Foundation in Ventura, California, and began in earnest to review and study the records of those who had for the prior twenty years been using movements like the cross-crawl as Brain Gym exercises. He concluded that Brain Gym exercises stimulate both the expressive (right) and receptive (left) hemispheres of the brain in order to advance integrated learning.

Dr. Dennison also developed his own techniques.

In order to get both your brain's hemispheres working in unison, try the following: March in place bringing the opposite arm and leg up simultaneously (cross-crawl). Once you feel comfortable with this, advance to a cross-crawl that requires alternating an arm and the opposite leg while humming and moving the eyes up, down, then to the left and the right. This can be done standing or lying down. The activity stimulates both brain hemispheres. Cross-crawl activities have been used for decades in neurological patterning to maximize learning potential. Experts believe that the contra-lateral movement activates the speech and language centers of the brain.

Spend a few minutes with this activity in the mornings and again in the evenings. Hum, don't sing words. Words require left-brain activity. You want to turn on both sides, not overload one side. If you have a stressful meeting with the boss, slip into the restroom and do a few cross-crawls to stabilize yourself, and make it easier for you to understand the logic and emotion of the situation.

You'll know the exercise is working if you feel more energetic, focused and coordinated. As such, it helps with everyday work and home activities. In addition it can facilitate time travel, for which you need the right-brain memory and the left-brain logic in order to understand what was happening and why. All the therapy sessions I conduct begin with this, because I want to work with a whole-brain client.

If you are homolateral, that is, oriented to one side of the brain, or if you have been in the military and marched with the same hand and foot moving together, you may need a therapist to retrain (re-pattern) the brain. We are born with the cross-crawl movement. It is innate but it becomes switched off due to emotional overloads, traumas, physical injuries and a host of other reasons.

Whole-brain integration can be helped along by other physical exercises, too, such as walking and swimming, where one arm and the opposite leg move. It is often while walking or running that people begin thinking and getting in touch. These whole-brain activities help open the memory bank.

Basic acupressure

Here is another technique which can be helpful, particularly in the release of false beliefs resulting from past trauma. This one involves the neurovascular points, which are located on the forehead halfway between the hairline and the eyebrow. Acupressure on these points, by the way, has a direct influence on the flow of energy throughout the body, according to the oriental science of meridians. A Chinese physician can detect imbalances in meridians by feeling pulses in more than five hundred different points on the body.

Hold these neurovascular points until you feel the pressure inside your head diminish. The sensation I experience is as though the blood flowing to my head begins returning to my stomach.

It may seem odd, but apparently there is a connection between these points and the stomach. Dr. John Thie, in his book *Touch for Health,* explains how to hold them until emotional stress no longer affects the abdomen. You can hold your own points, or someone else can hold them for you. We tend to hold stress in this part of our body, resulting in stomachaches or nervous stomachs. Holding the neurovascular points brings energy to the frontal lobes, where rational thought is available, without a negative emotional overlay. The natural response to stress, the "fight or flight" response, is alleviated, leaving room for a new response to be learned or activated.

People naturally use their neurovascular points, for example, when they put their hands on their foreheads after being told stress-inducing news. Rodin's statue The Thinker uses his hand on his chin to facilitate thought. He would find it easier if he would move his hand to his forehead to use his neurovascular points instead. The use of these points in a purposeful way can enhance your focus and bring peace to a volatile situation.

I often hold these points on my clients to help them replace old, limiting beliefs with new ones that will allow them to soar. During the silence I ask the clients to process the information deeply. Often they report that a vision appears concerning how what may have been troubling them will work out.

Spiritual music

Let's move on to accelerated learning techniques. These can be used to tap into memory stores that stem from our very beginning as spirits. Although we have known of the therapeutic value of classical music for centuries, it has only been recently that classical music has been used to help people memorize new languages, increase vocabulary and accelerate learning of other kinds. Music has a profound impact on the body, mind and soul. The pioneering work of the renowned Bulgarian psychiatrist George Lazanov, M.D., has brought us amazing new insights. Apparently, certain classical music can enhance learning by helping people relax, thereby heightening their ability to store information. Studies show that children who have music as part of their preschool curriculum perform better as students later than their peers who were not exposed to music lessons.

One way I have found to open up the memory bank through music is the Musical Body Program, which is available under the trademark TheraSound. Each of seven tapes in a different key creates a deep state of relaxation that helps unite the body and the mind. The rhythmic patterns and frequencies help the listener slow the rate of breath, release tension and focus thoughts and energy. When body and mind are calm, then thought, emotion and memory flow more freely. This, in turn, combats stress.

The Musical Body Program can be used as an adjunct therapy to help discover the root cause of a client's condition. It also can help remove blockages in the person's bio-energetic system and, thus, bring the client closer to his or her true nature. I sometimes use the tapes while giving a client new beliefs to replace old, destructive ones. They can be used by you at home.

A premise of using this music is that each of the seven chakras, or energy centers, vibrates at an optimum or healthy frequency. Each tape is specially designed to assist a particular chakra. For example, Tape #1 is the key of C, which resonates the base of the spine. In addition to dealing with lower back pain, the key of C helps to develop a strong identity and sense of purpose and the experience of being "grounded." The listener becomes more aware of taking responsibility for creating his or her life, according to the deepest understanding of what it means to be human. The deep relaxation and heightened awareness that result can stir up memories of the distant past.

While we are on the subject of tapes, Silva Method tapes are a way of gaining access to the alpha level of brain frequency, between seven and fourteen pulsations per second, in order to tap the powers of the right hemisphere. With their aid, the listener learns how to relax and to enter the alpha state. There are other tapes that resonate with the frequencies of an alpha state. A listener enters the alpha state simply by listening.

Music, memory and accelerated learning are interconnected, just as the body, mind and spirit are interconnected. Sickness in the body often affects how a person perceives herself and vice versa. If you think of getting a disease, you can actually create it. Hence, the term psychosomatic illness. Accelerated learning techniques use the most positive dimensions of this circular connection of body, mind and spirit.

Daily meditation

Perhaps more than any other, a technique that has been practiced for millennia, daily meditation can be one of the most powerful. It can connect you directly to the higher power within. As a result, what you need to work on can come to you. Memories of past lives also may be revealed, along with their deeper meaning.

Meditation may be practiced at any time, but for best results I suggest twice a day — in the morning when you first awake and in the evening before bed. Spend at least ten minutes and up to a half hour. I also find it helpful to take short meditation breaks throughout the day, especially when things get hectic.

Meditation techniques vary, but their general goal is to free a person of the illusions and noise of the world. It requires silence, an act of will, to enter the channel of Divine Knowing leading to the Divine Source.

In *Legacy of the Heart: The Spiritual Advantages of a Painful Childhood,* Wayne Muller recommends a useful exercise. Go to a quiet place, perhaps your personal refuge. Relax. Take time to breath deeply. Then softly say these words to yourself:

May I dwell in the heart.
May I be healed.
May I be filled with love.
May I be free from suffering.
May I be happy.
May I be at peace. (p.72)

This particular meditation derives from the Buddhist practice of metta, in which loving kindness is sent to all beings who inhabit the earth. Metta is like giving flowers to others: You cannot help but breathe in some of the fragrance yourself. As the practice of positive thinking grows within, you will create a better environment in which to cradle your soul. Once your soul feels safe and protected, it will permit you to remember. It will do so when you are ready, and can trust you not to abuse it or misuse the information.

Meditation is akin to prayer. Prayer is the act of asking for help from a higher being. True prayer is giving up your own will and asking the Divine Will to take over. For some, prayer is a wish list, as if God was a heavenly Santa Claus. But true prayer is deeper and more spiritual. Like meditation it is communion with a higher power.

In some cases prayer is a call for a past-life remembrance, though the person may not actually intend it that way. In Mary's case, the sorrow of her heart was the call. Since the call compels the answer, the person praying has to provide some way for the answer to come. The answer may be meditation. It may come when an individual is working with a therapist or reading a self-help book or attending a workshop. There are many traditional and non-traditional techniques being developed to match different learning styles. Many are the vehicles for the prayers of those who ask to be answered. Be alert to what seems to work best for you.

Often the past comes back in bits and pieces. Only after a-while will you have enough information and enlightenment to understand what it has to teach. This process can take months or even years. Indeed, it may take a lifetime if your inner child is fearful of exploration. There are several things you can do to reduce or eliminate fear and to stimulate the whole-brain activity that improves memory.

Maintain a journal

It is important to make a daily record of events and of your thoughts concerning them. You might also use journaling to record ideas or impressions that come to you while in meditation. Reading these later can stimulate valuable insights that may have been missed when they first occurred. Perhaps you were too close to events, too emotionally involved.

Often the insights come in a flash of understanding. You might be occupied in something as mundane as washing the dishes. All of sudden an image may come to you. Do not dismiss it. Rather, write it down and thank the universe for sending it. You have honored the gift and the giver. When you do this, more images will come. Mary wrote down her insights. By writing a journal she helped open the channel of remembering.

Visualization exercises

Your imagination also can be used for time travel. Two useful methods are "making a movie" and "entering a time machine." As you may remember, my clients Jim and Tom both made movies to help them move through the pain of an experience identified in age regression. Movies also enabled them to take on higher beliefs and to see from a broader perspective the events they needed to deal with.

The movie technique uses eye movements to trigger different parts of the brain. The following is a typical session that I as a therapist might have with a client.

> *Therapist:* I want you to close your eyes and keep them closed during this process. I'm going to tell you to move your eyes in various directions. Keep your eyelids closed while you do this. Are you ready? OK. Move your eyes

down and to the right. Now, I want you to make a movie of the situation that gave you so much stress. See the situation as it happened. See yourself doing just what you did then. Allow yourself to feel whatever you felt. When you are through, put your hands in your lap.

(Client completes instructions.)

Therapist: Move your eyes down and to the center, and run the same movie. This time, however, run it faster. See yourself doing the same things you did before, only faster. When you are done, unfold your hands.

(Client completes instructions.)

Therapist: Move your eyes down and to the left, and run the same movie as fast as you can. When you are done, fold your hands in your lap.

(Client completes instructions.)

Therapist: Turn your eyes up and to the right. Take three deep breaths and tell me what comes to your mind.

(Client writes down the comments. They will be brief and quick.)

Therapist: Turn your eyes up and to the center. Take two deep breaths and tell me what comes to your mind.

(Client does so.)

Therapist: Turn your eyes up and to the left. Take one deep breath and tell me what comes to your mind.

If the comments are positive, the session is finished; the goal has been reached. If the comments are negative or non-committal, continue in this way . . .

Therapist: Turn your eyes to the right ear and tell me what comes to you.

(Client does so.)

Therapist: Turn your eyes to the left ear and tell me what comes to you.

(Client does so.)

Therapist: Turn your eyes up and to the center, and check out your body. Notice if there is any pain, stress or tightness in any place in your body. When you find it, cause it to move to the top of your head. Imagine that above your head is an angel with a vacuum cleaner. The vacuum cleaner looks like a special model with a huge bag to hold all the stress. Let the stress go into the angel's vacuum cleaner.

As you release the negative feelings from the top of your head, begin to think that if the angel is going to take those feelings, why not also let her have all the tightness in your body.

Go to the tips of your toes and let all that stress come up through your body. Let it pull up the tightness from the toes, from the calves, up to the hips, the stomach, the back, the chest, the arms, the neck, up through the face and out the top of your head into the cosmic vacuum cleaner that now looks more like a hot air balloon.

Let the cosmic angel take the hot air balloon. It's now filled with all that stress and tightness; let the angel take it far away into the Universe to the Great Central Sun. The heat of the Great Central Sun bursts the balloon and changes the stress into snowflakes of beautiful colors. Pinks, golds, light blues. These snowflakes are love, wisdom and healing. They float down into your body through the top of your head, down through your neck, back, stomach and down into the very tips of your toes.

Now, as you sit here, the air is filled with snowflakes. Pink for love, yellow for wisdom, green for healing and prosperity. You are filled with peace, joy, understanding and love.

Your body is now filled with love. You may open your eyes whenever you are ready.

(End of session.)

The movie's purpose is to permit an individual to react less personally to a situation by moving through it, first at the normal speed, then faster and faster. The goal is detachment. As a person gets far enough away emotionally she sees events in a different light. She is able to create and see a bigger picture. Too often we take so much responsibility for a particular event that in a sense we become the event. As Zig Ziegler says, "Failure is an event. Not a person." Movies help us see the situation in a different way, less emotionally and with more logic.

During the movie, especially when the eyes are up, a person develops insight. Insight increases the more relaxed the individual allows herself to be. Once she makes the picture bigger, this new reality will stay with her. When the old stresses are cleared away, the inner child has more energy to explore the past, because it knows that no harm will come as it remembers.

Let's discuss what I call the Time Machine.

This technique uses progressive relaxation. A person begins by counting backwards or tightening the muscles of her body, one by one, and then releasing each tightened muscle until the entire body is relaxed.

As a therapist, I might say softly, "Tighten the muscles in the eyes. Tighten them even more. Now, release and feel the difference. Feel the lightness. Now, tighten the muscles in the eyes again. Feel the hardness. Tighten harder. Now, release and feel the relaxation. Welcome it."

Once you have discovered how to tighten and release the muscles that surround your eyes, move to the jaw. Then the neck muscles, the hand, the biceps by making a fist and tightening the whole arm. Continue with any and all muscles of the body down to the feet, or until you are aware you might go to sleep.

Once your body is more relaxed, imagine taking an elevator down into the depth of your being, where there is a special room. Decorate this room in any way that is comfortable for you. Then go over to a special machine, a time machine. Place your hand on the control that will move you through time — forward or backwards.

Let me interject that the first time you do this, you may want to be in the presence of another person who is trained or experienced enough to help. If you see something too upsetting when you go back into the past, you might want someone there to help comfort you or to debrief you when you return.

When you wish to return to the present, leave the room and come back up the elevator. Upon returning, it is important to thank the giver of the information. And remember, you have been to that private room; it is yours and you can always return. Anytime you wish.

Devotionals

The *violet flame affirmation technique* taught by Saint Germain is another way to transmute past events without having to go through the pain of remembering. It is a very powerful use of the principle of the spoken word and a violet ray of light. The violet light serves as a flame to burn through the cause and core of the memory, and thus dissolve it forever.

Saint Germain was a fascinating individual. He dazzled the

royal courts of eighteenth century Europe in an attempt to avert the bloody French Revolution and earned the name, "Wonder Man of Europe." It has been documented that he transmuted flaws in diamonds, disappeared into thin air and spoke many languages while at the French royal court. He is credited with having expanded scientific knowledge to fan the flame of the Industrial Revolution. This master "alchemist" was, however, seen by those in power as more of an entertainer than a "master of self." Thus, he did not gain a large following, and his goal went unrealized of creating a republican form of "God-over-men" (government). His dream that the God-identity would be in every person's heart in France failed, and instead, the French Revolution prevailed.

The French and other Europeans did not realize that in fact St. Germain was an ascended being. He earned his ascension by making over two million right choices in his own progress of mastery over self. After his ascension he was given a special chance to return in a physical body to assist his brothers and sisters to move higher in consciousness.

Today Saint Germain is considered Master of the Seventh Ray and Master of the Aquarian Age. One of his greatest teachings has to do with the "violet flame." It acts as a cosmic cleaner, sucking up the debris in a person's life and in the world, permitting the reversal of the misuse of God's energy.

Violet flame decrees are affirmations, but they are also much more. Affirmations and decrees use the power of the vibration of sound expressed as a word. Words form pictures that stay in our minds. ("Thoughts are things.") The word "geometry," for example, is said by some to have a deeper meaning. The G stands for God, being life and light. The E stands for energy. The OM stands for the sound chanted by Buddhist monks, the perfect sound, "AUUMM." This utterance contains all the vowel sounds and, thus, at least a particle of every word in every language. It communicates God's light (His Word) and belief in the ability to create life. Thus, creation is geometric (2 x 2 = 4; 4 x 4 = 16, et cetera), instead of arithmetical (1 + 1 = 2; 2 + 2 = 4). In this way words become "works"— mind pictures or constructions.

Each word might be likened to a chalice. Each contains a certain power of vibration. An opera singer, for example, can shatter a goblet by sounding a particular pitch. Native American shamans use "toning" to heal. Decrees combine the vibration of words in combination with others to develop momentum or cadence.

Words are powerful because they convey thoughts. The Gospel of John, for example, referred to God as the Word. ("And the Word became flesh.") God is the Word, and Christ is the flesh. Affirmations such as those used by Christ can be decrees. For example, Jesus, the Christ, used these words: "I AM the Light, the Truth and the Way." You might affirm this by saying: "I AM Light, Light, Light."

Notice what happens when you invoke light within yourself. If you see the light as bright, energizing, consuming all your darkness, you will feel lighter. If you think of light as murky, intermittent, you will feel that instead of the intensity of the power of bright light.

Given how we see in our minds what we are saying with our words, the power of the decree is not just in the combination of the words that form the cadence. Thoughts evoked and the thrust from the heart make a spoken word like a sword, or a laser beam to cut through what should not be.

Decrees are edicts. They are what caused the walls of Jericho to fall. They are used as authoritative decisions (a divorce decree, for example). They are also commands. In the Book of Job (22:28) it says, "Thou shalt decree a thing, and it shall be established unto thee: and the light shall shine upon thy ways." Thus, Jesus, the Christ, stilled the troubled waters by saying, "Peace. Be still and know that I AM God."

When the spoken word is combined with a desire in our heart and sent into the Universe on a particular ray of light, the message becomes like a radio or TV wave. You are created in God's image. Just as God spoke the world into being, you can create that which you desire.

The pink wave of light is often used for the sounds and words of love. Pink conjures up images of Cupid and hearts. As a matter of contrast, imagine the tune that is played at high school graduations called "Pomp and Circumstance." It would be seen as a blue wave of power and God's will.

Each ray of light has a special frequency, power and purpose. The violet ray is the ray of transmutation, changing both the giver of the decree and that which the decreer desires to be changed. It is a FORGIVENESS ray. As a person says violet flame decrees, he or she becomes the violet flame in action. She becomes a balance of the power and fire of the Old Testament and the love and compassion of the New.

In *Violet Flame to Heal the Body, Mind and Spirit*, Elizabeth Clare Prophet explains the many uses of the violet flame. In the final chapter of her book are several very simple decrees such as "I AM a being of Violet Fire." You may wish to get a copy and use these degrees. Tapes are also available that can help a person incorporate the use of this very powerful technique into one's life.

Like angels, prayer and meditation, the violet flame is a free gift to us all regardless of our religious affiliation. Saint Germain through the Theosophical society, the I AM Movement and the books written by Godfrey Ray King such as *Unveiled Mysteries,* all have laid the foundation for our present knowledge and use of violet flame decrees.

When I first started using this technique, I would think about the situations such as crime, drug dealing and violence that I wanted to decrease, have consumed and have taken from this planet. Then I would imagine putting those challenges into the violet flame and say with love in my heart, "I AM the violet flame in action in me now, I AM the violet flame to Light alone I bow."

These decrees are not vain repetitions — not if you use your mind and see the flame consuming problems, and you are centered in your heart and not aiming to inflict pain upon others.

When I say a decree, I experience an immediate spiritual uplift. After fifteen minutes I feel better about myself and my affairs, and I have more energy. After six months of doing fifteen minutes of decrees daily, I was able to see significant changes in the world around me and in my relationships.

The decree may be short or long. It is usually preceded by a formal preamble and a closing or acceptance. As you burn off the "density" in and around you, your third eye will open to spiritual matters. And to the past.

The preamble is like an opening to a prayer where special masters are invoked for favors, such as the following:

> Expand the Violet Flame within my heart; purify my body; transmute all disqualified energy I have ever imposed upon life; and blaze mercy's healing ray throughout the earth, the elementals and all mankind, and answer this my call, infinitely, presently and forever.

The closing can be a simple, "Amen."

Now that you are more willing to accept the responsibility of remembering the past, what happens if you do have a remembrance of something from another place and time? How can this information from the past help with the present?

Always keep in mind that the purpose of remembering is to make us more aware of what we need to deal with, learn and perhaps exorcise in order to live our divine plan for this life. If we are carrying around excess baggage, the best thing we can do is unload it. Clean out the attic. Not to do so is to allow ourselves to continue in pain instead of peace, poverty instead of plenty, fear instead of love.

Loved ones who are patiently waiting beyond the veil pray for us to move more quickly, for it is easier and better to make the corrections we need to make now, while we are on this physical plane. There is an ultimate purpose to remembering, and we must begin to do so where we presently are.

Meditation

Visualize the still waters of the lake of peace. There is no movement except a gentle lapping of the water on the margin of the lake. Meditate by the shore of the lake and feel the cool, cleansing touch of the water upon your feet and hands and brow. All is so still . . .

There is a path of light across the surface of the water into the heart of the Sun . . . All that is of the earth in you, all that separates, is consumed in the light of the Sun.

Be still . . . in the Sun.

Source: The Still Voice, The White Eagle Publishing Trust, page 52.

CONCLUSION
HOW TO INTERPRET PAST LIFE MEMORIES

You may wish to get a notebook to record what you remember of a particular past experience. Because of the complexity and the emotions involved, it often is best that you write down the memories. Then you'll be ready to follow the five steps below. In doing so, you will become your own therapist.

1. Identify the participants or players. Are they males? Females?

2. Note what they are doing.

3. Come up with a set of belief statements that would support what they are doing.

4. Change the set of belief statements in Step three to a higher, positive set.

5. Replace the old belief system with the new one.

Let's look at each step for greater clarity.

1. Identify the participants or players.

Do this as you would for dream analysis. For the purposes of this work, the players are symbolic characters. They are our mirrors, reflecting back to us the male and female aspects of our being. We need the separate males and females to act out the parts, to be our teachers, showing us the gaps in our being in order to integrate these aspects.

In Mary's memory King Arthur is a separate person. He also represents her male aspect. The queen is in reality another aspect of Mary, her female aspect.

2. *Note what they are doing.*

If it was good, then claim that strength. That good is one of the treasures stored in heaven that you can now claim because you passed the test once. You have a right to the treasure now.

Unfortunately, some of our greatest strength comes from decisions that left us feeling guilty. In our effort to deny that we can make poor choices, we rob ourselves of the strength by pushing the decision from our memory.

Most events have positive as well as stressful components. Even a horrific event, such as the one recounted in the introduction of this book of Pearl being raped at age eight by her father, had a positive element. Sometimes it is this hidden awareness that it is most important to bring to the forefront of consciousness. When my own therapist would say, "More stress," I was pushed to remember the most critical parts. Be willing to explore deeply. Remember, though, that what does not come up this time may come up later in another session, when you are more willing to accept responsibility for your part in an event.

3. *Come up with a belief system that would support what they are doing.*

Ask yourself, "What could a person be believing to act that way?" Remember that people go to great lengths to justify their belief systems, even those that are not in their best interest.

Mary was the servant to both the king and the queen. She must have believed that she had to be a servant. In her present life if being a servant for a low wage is not what she wants, she needs a new belief statement to replace the old. With a new belief statement she will attract the new situation that will prove her belief statement to be true.

There was a war in Mary's past life. She did not believe in war per se, but rather that human sacrifice was necessary to attain freedom. That belief served her well in those days. Today, however, it is important for her and us to stay in the body, rather than to sacrifice our bodies in an effort to be free. The spirit combined with the physical body is a very powerful force, one that is needed to bring in the new millennium.

If you discover warring males in your past, it probably means that you are warring with your male aspect (and in some cases, several male aspects), regardless of whether you are presently embodied as a male or a female. Having warring females means you probably are not cooperating with your female aspect. Admit it. Forgive yourself and choose to be at peace.

4. Change the set of belief statements in Step Three to a higher, positive set.

Some things about the past experience should be taken literally. However, when the other person is male, you should conceive of the new belief in terms of a male aspect. For example, in the past life of Mary, King Arthur blamed himself for losing the battle. He assured all that it was his responsibility. King Arthur represents nothing more nor less than Mary's male aspect. Instead of saying, "King Arthur blames himself for losing the battle," the new belief would be, "My male aspect blames himself for losing the battle." That statement reflects the male aspect, but it is still negative.

An even higher, more positive statement would be, "My male aspect no longer blames himself for losing the battle. He no longer assumes all of the responsibility." Or, "Human sacrifice is no longer needed in order to attain freedom." We change the negative belief statement into a positive one in order to move from the past into the future.

One of the most powerful, new belief statements may be, "My male aspects are no longer emotionally abusive."

Don't be confused because the statement above uses a plural for the male aspect. We may be one individual but have many inner children, and thus have male aspects at different ages. With male and female aspects working together, you can now attract to yourself a beloved one who will honor his own feminine and masculine aspects as well as yours. There is a greater chance for peace and harmony in a relationship that increases the spirituality of both. Key words in a new statement are "no longer" or "now," such as, "I now work cooperatively and peacefully with my male aspects."

Create statements that turn the stressful into the positive may begin with:

"Now I am . . . "

"Now I am a miracle, and miracles are happening through me."

"Now I am confident in all situations."

"Now I am kindness."

"Now I am deserving of and receptive to kindness."

To deal specifically with the male and female aspects, the statements might begin with, "Now my male aspect is..."

"Now my male aspect is supportive of my growth and development."

"Now my female aspect loves and approves of me."

"Now my male and female aspects are communicating with each other."

You can muscle-test yourself to see if your muscles are still weak when this new statement is said. The objective is for your muscles to remain strong, which indicates the new belief system has taken hold.

Most of the time I work on the statements that produce weakness in my muscles. If you test strong in a belief statement, it may not need attention. But then again, it might. For example, Jim, the basketball player, was strong in his belief, "I am alone." What he really wanted, however, was a special love. He would either have to give up his conflicting desire for love or give up on the belief statement. Always consider the consequences that might flow from a new belief statement or system before you proceed.

5. Replace the old belief system with the new one.

Replacement strategies include making movies, holding the vascular points on the head, verbalizing and simply realizing that there is a higher way. I determine the best course through muscle-testing. In this way an individual's higher self tells me what technique will work best. Sometimes, it is a prayer we give together. Sometimes, it is my leaving the client in silence for several minutes, so his or her own spiritual essence can rekindle memory.

Sometimes, we have a celebration.

"What would you do," I ask, "to celebrate if these statements were true for you?"

Some take themselves and their loved ones out to dinner or go to the park for a long walk. You will know what you need to affirm these new statements.

What once brought weakness and stress is now a strength. Watch as your life changes for the better. If you had a critical mother in your past, it is usually because your own female aspect does not have a belief system that includes, "My female aspect loves and approves of me." As you become more loving to your female aspect, you will find your relationship with your mother improving. It works almost like magic. It is truly brought about by divine inspiration.

It is your own belief system, brimming with emotion and sent out as thoughts into the Universal Mind, that attracts others of like mind and being to you. If you do not like what is around you, you can change your belief system and thereby begin to broadcast different thoughts that will attract newcomers with the gentle and loving aspects that you seek.

Truly, you create your own world. Through remembrance, you erase and replace the beliefs that caused errors and hardship in the past. You can also claim the good and the strength of what has gone before. In so doing, you will create a future that can be a heaven on earth.

In closing, I want to share my first past life experience using kinesiology/ results techniques as a therapist. It was conducted under the direction of my teacher. In fact, a number of therapists were in training together. My teacher teamed me with a very tall, heavy man, who had a head as bald as Kojack's. My assignment was to play the role of the therapist. His was to be the client.

He made himself calm and became quiet as instructed. I began working with his fingers. We identified the need for him to experience a time and place in his mind before this time, in order to deal with whatever was at the root of the emotional stress in his life. I asked him to become like an angel on a cloud, a spirit without a body. I asked him to return to a time and place that would come to him, a time and place that he wanted or needed to revisit. Perhaps it was a time that had always fascinated him.

As he became quiet, I was able to tune into his frequency. It was as if we were one, each and both seeking healing.

His eyes were closed. Mine were open so that I could record what he said. He began seeing himself in the Old West with the Indians. He described how he trapped for the skins of animals. He described how it was done, how the animals were mistreated and wasted. Then he began to talk about how he killed Indians, as though they, too, were nothing more than animals. As he spoke, my eyes filled with tears. I experienced deep sorrow for my brothers as he explained how he had scalped them.

He continued to talk about how the scalping was done, and I continued to feel the pain of my ancestors, to be drawn deeper and deeper into sorrow. Finally, I'd had about all that I could stand. I wanted to stand up and run. I wanted to leave that place, to quit that session.

Then all at once, a strange feeling came over me. Suddenly, I felt compassion for this big bald man, as though a voice were saying that it was now my role to extend forgiveness. I, as a descendent of Native Americans, had been chosen as a representative of my race. This man had done those acts in ignorance. The truth was that his heart was really as big as his body.

I was transformed by this session, and so was the big bald man. Today he will not destroy any living thing. Not even a fly. It would be contrary to his new belief system.

I was healed, and he was healed.

You see, I was in as much need of healing of those wounds as he had been for inflicting them. Each of us required forgiveness for the parts we had played in causing pain and anguish for the other. For when we come to the center of our being, we are love compassion, joy, hope and forgiveness.

So, as you use these techniques to heal, prepare for miracles. They will come, both to you and others. Once you acquire insight from past memories and incorporate the lesson they have to teach, you will be ready to experience a future perhaps never before imagined. As you have traveled to the past, so will you travel to the future. You will ascend to ever higher levels of understanding and achievement. Ultimately, in this, or a future time mastery will be yours.

Toward that goal, and in all your travels, I wish you God-speed.

I want to say something to all of you who have become
a part of the fabric of my life.

The color and texture which you have brought into my being
have become a song and I want to sing it forever.

There is an energy in us which makes things happen
when the path of other persons touch ours, and we have
to be there and let it happen.

When the time of our particular sunset comes, our thing,
our accomplishments won't really matter a great deal.

But the clarity and care with which we have loved
others will speak with vitality of the great gift we have
been for each other.

—The Monks of Weston Priory

NOTES